Cognitive-Communicative Abilities Following Brain Injury

A Functional Approach

Neurogenic Communication Disorders Series

SERIES EDITOR

Leonard L. LaPointe, Ph.D.

Cognitive-Communicative Abilities Following Brain Injury

A Functional Approach

Leila L. Hartley, Ph.D.
Director of Staff Development
Transitional Learning Community at Galveston
Galveston, Texas

S SINGULAR PUBLISHING GROUP, INC.
SAN DIEGO, CALIFORNIA

Singular Publishing Group, Inc.
4284 41st Street
San Diego, California 92105-1197

© 1995 by Singular Publishing Group, Inc.

Typeset in 10.5/12.5 Goudy Oldstyle by House Graphics
Printed in the United States of America by McNaughton & Gunn

Library of Congress Cataloging-in-Publication Data

Hartley, Leila L.
  Cognitive Communicative abilities following brain injury : a
functional approach / Leila L. Hartley.
        p.   cm. — (Neurogenic communication disorders series)
    Includes bibliographical references and index.
    ISBN 1-56593-102-5
    1. Brain damage—Patients—Rehabilitation.   2. Cognition
disorders—Patients—Rehabilitation.   3. Language disorders—
Patients—Rehabilitation.   I. Title.   II. Series.
    [DNLM: 1. Brain Injuries—rehabilitation.   2. Communicative
Disorders—therapy.   3. Cognition.   4. Social Adjustment.   WL 354
H332c 1994]
    RC387.5.H37 1994
    616.85'503—dc20
    DNLM/DLC
    for Library of Congress   94-28243
                                                                              CIP

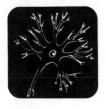

Contents

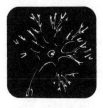

Foreword

The brain is a marvelous thing. It has been called the only human organ capable of studying itself. Although the metaphoric heart has been rhapsodized in song and sonnet much more frequently, the brain and its peculiar music have met increasing attention, not only popularly, but notably from researchers, scholars, educators, and clinicians who must deal with attempts to understand it. In fact, in the United States, the commitment to understanding the brain and its disorders has been reflected in the highest policy levels of the government, and the White House Office of Science and Technology Policy focused this attention in a report entitled "Maximizing Human Potential: Decade of the Brain 1990-2000."

When the human nervous system goes awry, the cost is enormous. Direct and indirect economic impact of brain disorders in the United States has been estimated to be over $400 billion. It is impossible to measure the toll that brain disorders extract in terms of human agony from victims and their families. Each disruption of delicate neural balance can cause problems in moving, sensing, eating, thinking, and a rich array of human behaviors. Certainly not the least of these are those unique human attributes involved in communication. To speak, to understand, to write, to read, to remember, to create, to calculate, to plan, to reason . . . and myriad other cognitive and communicative acts are the sparks and essence of human interaction. When they are lost or impaired, isolation can result, or at the very least, quality of life can be compromised. This series is about those many conditions that arise from brain or nervous system damage that can affect these human cognitive and communicative functions. But it is not only an attempt to understand the disruption and negative effects of neurogenic disorders. As well, the authors in this series will show that there is a positive side. Rehabilitation, relearning, intervention, recovery, adjustment, acceptance, and reintegration are the rewards to be extracted from challenge. There will be no shortage of these features in this series. Frustrations and barriers can be redeemed by recovery and small victories. The words in this Singular Series on Neurogenic Communication Disorders address both the obstacles and the triumphs.

The big book of words, *The Random House Dictionary of the English Language (Unabridged)* defines "functional" as *of or pertaining to the kind of action or activity proper to a person, thing, or institution; the purpose for which something is designed or exists.* When the tragedy of traumatic brain injury occurs, the person affected encounters unprecedented challenge in achieving the proper activities of living, learning, and loving. The quiet epidemic of brain injury has spread its tentacles into all aspects of modern society, but most prodigiously among young people from mid-teens to mid-twenties. Brain injury has a significant effect not only on the person devastated by a car crash, but predictably on the immediate family. The community as a whole is affected by the drains placed on its financial and rehabilitation resources. Although increasing attention is apparent in the literature on the neuropathophysiology and behavioral sequelae of shattered cortex and brain stem, very little guidance is available on routes of recovery.

This book by Leila L. Hartley offers a distinctive and applicable approach to rehabilitation of the crushing cognitive-communicative deficits that follow brain injury. Dr. Hartley brings a rich clinical and scholarly experience to the disorder. I had the pleasure of working with her during her doctoral training at the University of Florida. She came to us from a large rehabilitation hospital where she was responsible for evaluation and treatment of a demanding caseload of individuals with brain injury. Since those days she has enhanced her adroitness by layer upon layer of research and clinical interaction. As will be apparent from this book, she has developed a philosophy for dealing with the cognitive-communicative deficits to be remediated, and this approach is firmly grounded in all that is meant by the term "functional." Dr. Hartley believes that assessment and treatment are best aimed at daily living issues, that is, the development of self-regulatory skills and compensatory strategies that can be integrated into functional environments. She has unfolded these approaches clearly and with sound rationale in this book. I have no doubt that it will prove to be a functional treasure for professionals and families faced with the struggle of brain injury.

Leonard L. LaPointe, Ph.D.
Series Editor
Arizona State University

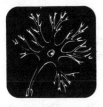

Preface

Brain injury rehabilitation is a relatively new field that has been full of challenges and changes since its conception. This is particularly so at the postacute level of rehabilitation. At this stage of recovery, the focus is on reestablishing on individual's meaningful relationships, restoring daily living skills, and rebuilding a productive lifestyle, despite any residual cognitive, communicative, and physical limitations. This level of rehabilitation generally follows a medical rehabilitation or inpatient rehabilitation phase and is provided in either a residential program, day program, or outpatient program aimed at community reintegration. This stage of rehabilitation emphasizes the strengths of an individual and the ability of the individual to learn new skills and strategies that will improve everyday functioning.

All rehabilitation services may aspire to reach functional outcomes, but the achievement of functional outcomes is the heart and soul of postacute rehabilitation. This is a tremendous challenge when working with individuals with traumatic brain injury because the needs of these individuals are so vast, yet so diverse. In addition, the potential for functional gains over a long period of time has to be balanced against the demand for reduced lengths of stay and greater cost effectiveness by funding sources.

This book seeks to identify a systematic approach for addressing the cognitive-communicative needs of individuals with traumatic brain injury at the postacute stage of rehabilitation. The emphasis in this book is on the communication aspect of cognitive-communicative functioning. There have been a number of books written to address cognitive rehabilitation, but few that have given more than cursory attention to communication.

This book provides a theoretical perspective for understanding social communication and a methodology for defining socially relevant goals for cognitive-communicative intervention. Two major themes dominate the text—maximizing social competency and rebuilding functional life skills.

Although the major focus of this book is dealing with the constellation of symptoms found after closed head injury, the approaches proposed are applicable to a broad range of communicative disorders, including those from cerebrovascular accident, anoxia, or infectious disease, as well as language and learning problems in adolescence. Furthermore, the methods for clinical practice advocated in this book are felt to be applicable to all rehabilitation disciplines, despite the author's background in speech-language pathology.

Throughout the book, the need for a coordinated, integrated, interdisciplinary—if not transdisciplinary— approach is underscored. Consistency of effort is necessary to effect clinical changes in cognitive-communicative abilities with this population. At this stage of rehabilitation, the active participation of the individual as well as the family is also of immense importance. Only through honest, open communication between all players—the clinical team, the individual, the family, other persons of particular significance to the individual served, and the funding source representative—can realistic, yet meaningful, outcomes be identified, targeted, and achieved.

It should be pointed out that careful attention has been given to the selection of terminology in this book to demonstrate sensitivity to the dignity and rights of the persons served in rehabilitation. To prevent the connotation of a subservient role for the person with brain injury, the terms *individual* or *individual with brain injury* are used throughout the book rather than *patient* or *client*. In addition, phrases such as *victims of brain injury* or *suffered a head injury* have been avoided because the terms interfere with expectations of preserved capability and empowerment. Furthermore, the words *deficits* and *weaknesses* are avoided and replaced with the terms *needs* or *challenges*, whenever possible.

This book attempts to balance theory and practice. Clinical practices must be based on a strong, sound, conceptual foundation; it is hard to plot a route when the destination and purpose are unknown. This book does not have all the answers regarding cognitive-communicative abilities following brain injury. Hopefully, however, clinicians will find some degree of guidance for increasing the social competence and functional life skills of individuals with brain injury.

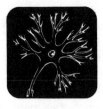

Acknowledgments

This book is a product of many years of clinical and research experience with individuals with brain injuries and an unending search for the most effective methods of intervention. The ideas are not all my own, but are synthesized from many sources. Much credit is given to the pioneers of functional assessment and brain injury rehabilitation.

I would like to acknowledge persons who have been instrumental in my professional growth and development. Special gratitude is expressed to Dr. Michelle Jensen and the late Dr. Paul Jensen, cherished mentors and friends who have encouraged, guided, and inspired me throughout my career. Much credit must be given as well to Dr. Leonard LaPointe. Without his editorial guidance and faith in my abilities, this book would not exist.

I would like to express my appreciation to all the trainees and staff of the Transitional Learning Community at Galveston, Texas. In my 9 years of employment there, I have had the opportunity to learn so much from these persons. The dedication, openness, competence, and creativity of its clinicians are unsurpassed. Its trainees have taught me much about courage and perseverance; the desire for a meaningful life; the value of life, love, and family; and what works and does not work in clinical practice. Their families have been incredible teachers, too, of what can be accomplished when all players work together, of the importance of family support, and of the need for greater community supports and options.

There are several persons from the Transitional Learning Community who deserve special recognition. I am immensely grateful to the administration for its support of this project. Dr. Brent Masel provided additional assistance through his careful review of the information on medications. Appreciation is sincerely expressed to Latasha Bellow for her endless hours of careful typing and proofing of the manuscipt. Additional assistance was provided by Georgina Eastmond. I also want to thank my colleagues, Dr. Monica McHenry and Rose Leal, for their assistance and encouragement.

The highest degree of gratitude is expressed to Robert L. Moody and The Moody Foundation of Galveston for their generous support for the preparation of this book (Moody Foundation Grant No. 91-29). Their advocacy efforts and generosity have tremendously advanced brain injury research and rehabilitation. Their devotion to this cause has inspired and improved the lives of so many persons with brain injury and their families. On a more personal level, I am extremely grateful for their support of my research and publication endeavors aimed at improving functional outcomes following brain injury.

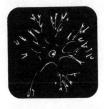

Dedication

To my husband, Jim, and daughter, Lindsey, for their patience, understanding, and love.

To my parents for their unending love and encouragement.

To Russell Moody for his humor, joy of life, persistence, and courage.

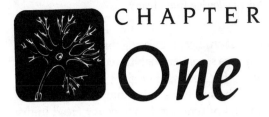

CHAPTER

One

Developing a Functional Perspective

Freeways accidents, assaults, domestic violence, work site accidents—read any newpaper and see how frequently these events are a part of today's world. In a fraction of a second, a person's mind can be altered forever. The tragedy of acquired brain injury is so pronounced because of its suddenness in the midst of typical development and because of its multiple long-term effects on the person, the family, and society as a whole. As stated by Harrison and Dijkers, "Injuries to the brain are one of the most catastrophic in terms of their numbers, severity, human suffering, economic loss and associated health care and related costs" (1992, p. 204).

Incidence of Brain Injuries and Risk Factors

Incidence of Traumatic Brain Injuries

Although it is clear that the incidence of traumatic brain injury (TBI) is of significant magnitude, the actual number of occurrences is difficult to ascertain. Incidence rates vary from study to study, because of differences in definitions of brain injury and in reporting procedures (Frankowski, Annegers, & Whitman, 1985; Harrison & Dijkers, 1992; Willer, Abosh, & Dahmer, 1990). Annual incidence rates of 200 brain injuries per 100,000

1

persons have been suggested by most studies, indicating that approximately 500,000 persons sustain brain injuries severe enough to require hospitalization each year in the United States (Frankowski et al., 1985; Interagency Head Injury Task Force, 1989). Of the survivors, it is estimated that 70,000 to 90,000 experience permanent loss of function (Interagency Head Injury Task Force, 1989). A study of unduplicated registry cases of live traumatic brain injury (TBI) hospital discharges in Florida, however, suggests an incidence rate of 70 per 100,000 population, with 21% of those cases exhibiting moderate to severe brain injuries (Hensley, 1988).

Neither incidence rate, however, likely accurately reflects the true rate of occurrences, because mild brain injuries are underreported; individuals not requiring hospitalization are not included in most registries or studies (Harrison & Dijkers, 1992). Only 50% (Frankowski et al., 1985) to 84% (Fife, 1987) of all cases of head injury are hospitalized. Nevertheless, evidence now demonstrates that even a mild brain injury, without loss of consciousness, can produce significant consequences (Barth et al., 1989; Bohnen, Twijnstra, & Jolles, 1992).

Causes of Brain Injury

Nationally, motor vehicle accidents are the number one cause of brain injury, accounting for 30 to 50% of all cases. The second leading cause is falls, explaining 20 to 30% of the cases of brain injury. The incidence of brain injury from interpersonal violence varies from 7% in more rural areas (Annegers, Grabow, Kurland, & Louis, 1980) to 40% in urban areas (Whitman, Coonley-Hoganson, & Desai, 1984).

Risk Factors

Epidemiological studies have identified risk factors associated with brain injuries. The risk is greatest in late adolescence or young adulthood, between the ages of 15 to 24 for males and 15 to 19 for females (Kraus, 1987). Additional peaks in incidence occur in the elderly population and in young childhood, with falls accounting for the majority of injuries. Males are not only two to three times as likely as females to sustain a brain injury but are also four to five times more likely to die when receiving a brain injury (Cooper et al., 1983; Frankowski et al., 1985). In addition, evidence exists for a relationship between low socioeconomic status or residence in high density urban areas and a higher incidence of brain injury (Axelrod, 1986; Fife, Faich, Hollinshead, & Boynton, 1986).

Additional factors that have been associated with increased risk for brain injury include substance abuse (Annegers et al., 1980; Sparadeo, Strauss, & Barth, 1990), preexisting learning disorder (Haas, Cope, & Hall, 1987), pretraumatic individual or family dysfunction or psychiatric illness (Rimel & Jane, 1984), and prior brain injury (Annegers et al., 1980; Salcido & Costich, 1992). In a study by Jagger, Levine, and Jane (1984), 31% of persons acutely hospitalized for brain injury reported a previous brain injury hospitalization.

Costs to Individual, Family, and Society

Faster and better emergency medical services, establishment of specialized trauma centers, and medical technological advances over the past 20 years have led to increased numbers of survivors of trauma. This means that many of the individuals who sustain even very severe brain injuries now survive with varying degrees of disability or changes in their quality of life. Consequently, the need for long-term, specialized rehabilitation programs; independent living programs; and other support services has greatly increased as individuals and families seek the highest degree of functional recovery possible.

The Monetary Costs of Brain Injury

The financial costs of a brain injury to an individual and to society are astounding. Lehmkuhl, Kreutzer, and Gordan (1992) report their preliminary findings from five model brain injury programs. Patients in their data bank on the average spent 28 days in an acute care hospital at an average daily cost of $2,305 for a total of $65,017 per individual and an additional 48 days in inpatient rehabilitation at an average cost of $1,096 a day for an additional $52,339 per individual. The rehabilitation and medical needs do not stop at inpatient rehabilitation, however. Although costs vary from case to case, total lifetime costs of care for a person with a severe brain injury have been estimated at $4.6 million (Deutsch, as reported in Noble, Conley, Laski, & Noble, 1990).

The tangible costs of brain injuries to society include not only costs for medical treatment and rehabilitation, but also social services for individuals and/or families and lost or reduced wages for the individuals and family members. Because of increased medical costs, increased numbers of survivors, and the increased length of rehabilitative services, overall monetary costs have been estimated to approach $25 billion annually (Interagency Head Injury Task Force, 1989).

The Human Cost

No monetary value can adequately reflect the devastating effects of brain injury on a person's life, as illustrated by the following examples.

Case 1. Pam was a beautiful, bright, blonde 19-year-old who was at a major turning point in her life; she had just graduated from high school and was preparing for fall admission to a Texas university. Although extremely close with her family, she and her parents were prepared for her upcoming move to college 500 miles away. Their lives were dramatically changed one day in June when a man ran a stop sign and plowed into the car Pam was driving. She was in a coma for 25 days. When she did emerge from coma, her physical recovery was slow but remarkable; she moved from wheelchair to walker by that December, from walker to quad cane by February, and from cane to unaided ambulation by 1 year postinjury. Her speech did not begin to return until 9 months postinjury, but became intelligible to familiar listeners in quiet settings by 1 year. Fortunately her memory, attention, judgment, and motivation were relatively intact. Her insight, however, was limited, and her concreteness and irritability resulted in tense social interactions and unrealistic goal setting. She had gaps in her knowledge base, reduced reading comprehension for college-level material, slowness in processing, and difficulty organizing her class notes and completing tests within the allotted time. Her ability to complete her goal of a college degree in journalism continues to be highly questionable after 2 years, and her awkward gait, tight left hand, and whisper-like speech are harsh, visible reminders of the accident to all who come in contact with her.

Case 2. Jack was a 30-year-old, third-year medical student who was an outstanding rugby player and professional cave diver. During a rugby match, he received a blow to his head that resulted in a right frontal subdural hematoma. Except for minor problems in his balance and a general "awkwardness," his motor skills were intact almost immediately. His behavior and social communication skills were on the surface good; he was polite, outgoing, generous, sociable, and likeable—just as friends reported him to be before his injury. His ability to regulate his thinking and social behavior, however, was significantly impaired, as indicated by reduced initiation of action, poor planning and follow-through of goal-directed activities, and impulsivity. In addition, his memory was not at its premorbid level. After a failed attempt at returning to medical school, he held a series of jobs, experiencing difficulty maintaining employment even as a laborer for a moving company.

The psychological toll of a brain injury on an individual is devastating. The injured person awakes from coma into a strange new world caused by an event for which there is no memory. One young female thought she had actually died and was in a funeral home because her first images after emerging from coma in the neurosurgical intensive care unit were of a dead, covered body being removed from a neighboring room and of the bouquets of flowers surrounding her bed.

After emerging from the fog of coma and posttraumatic amnesia, individuals face the stress of undergoing rehabilitation without the benefit of reliable predictions of the length of recovery or the future outcome for their efforts. They face being confronted with their deficits daily by professionals and family members without fully understanding their limitations themselves. They must often leave their familiar surroundings, friends, and family to receive services and are all too often stripped of any power of self-determination. The usual means of achieving a sense of self-worth through social role fulfillment and productive activities are not available. They are advised to forget their past ambitions and take an unplanned life path. The financial and legal ramifications of an accident can add to anxiety and sense of helplessness.

The Impact on Family

The impact of a brain injury on an individual's family is also immense. Family members are typically poorly prepared to deal with a sudden descent into the complex medical and rehabilitation world of brain injury. They are even less equipped to cope with the changes in their loved one, the disruption of their family life, the difficulty in accessing appropriate services, the pressures of financial strain, anxiety concerning the unknown future, and the complexity of legal problems (Camplair, Kreutzer, & Doherty, 1990; Oddy, Humphrey, & Uttley, 1978; Sbordone, 1984; Willer, Allen, Durnan, & Ferry, 1990). Moreover, their anxiety, distress, and depression may even increase with time, as they try to meet not only the long-term financial and daily living needs of the individual but also the social and recreational needs (Brooks, Campsie, Symington, Beattie, & McKinlay, 1986; Jacobs, 1988; Kozloff, 1987). Recent findings indicate that even the siblings of severely injured individuals experience a high degree of psychological distress, leading them to display cognitive and behavioral difficulties (Orsillo, McCaffrey, & Fisher, 1993). The needs of families are great and have only recently been considered and systematically explored in the United States (Camplair et al., 1990).

The Challenges of Brain Injury Rehabilitation

In response to the increased need for services for individuals with brain injuries and their families, dramatic growth has occurred in the health care system. During the 1980s, rehabilitation facilities and programs designed specifically for individuals with acquired brain injuries sprouted in almost every state and major city. Not only did the number of survivors of brain injury increase, but also the scope and duration of rehabilitative services.

It is now generally recognized that individuals with brain injuries have the potential to recover over a longer period of time as compared to those with spinal cord injuries or cerebrovascular accidents (Cope, 1990). In addition, there is a greater awareness that many persons require postacute rehabilitation (rehabilitation after acute inpatient rehabilitation) before achieving successful reintegration into home, community, and work/school responsibilities and activities.

The rapid increase in brain injury programs has meant increased job opportunities for rehabilitation professionals. Individuals with brain injuries, however, present a challenge to even seasoned professionals for a number of reasons.

Heterogeneity of Individuals and Their Outcomes

A major reason why individuals with brain injuries present challenges is the extraordinary range of sequelae and complex needs within this population. The functional outcome for persons who survive brain injuries varies from lifelong institutionalization to return to an independent, productive life—perhaps with minor quality of life changes. This heterogeneity is due to an interaction of a number of variables that contribute to the consequences of brain injury. As illustrated in Figure 1–1, these factors include the preinjury characteristics of the individual, the effects of the injury, the individual's reaction to the changes, the physical and social environment, and the recovery, adaptation, or rehabilitation following the injury.

Injury Factors

A major factor in the relatively unique status of each individual with brain injury is the variety of pathophysiological mechanisms that contribute to brain injury location and severity. Traumatic brain injuries are classified as either a penetrating brain injury, generally a stab or gunshot wound, or a nonmissile or closed head injury. Individuals with missile or penetrating brain injuries generally sustain primarily focal lesions and therefore present a clearer clinical profile. On the other hand, individuals who have sustained nonpenetrating injuries or closed head injuries present a more complicated clinical symptomology and are the focus of this book.

The neuropathology of closed head injury, as outlined in Table 1–1, is the combined result of both primary and secondary brain injury (Graham, Adams, & Gennarelli, 1987). "Primary injury occurs immediately following impact and is related to instantaneous events directly caused by the blow" (Pang, 1985, p. 4). Secondary damage, on the other hand, is the result of pathologic processes that are the body's response to the primary damage. These complications do not present clinically immediately at the time of injury (Graham et al., 1987).

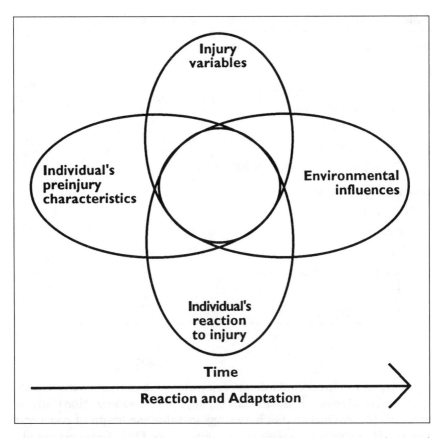

Figure 1-1. Factors contributing to the heterogeneity of symptomatology and outcomes after brain injury.

Both focal and diffuse brain injury are produced when blunt head trauma occurs. Focal injury is common at the site of the impact, as the skull bends inward from the force, as well as at the point directly opposite this site (known as coup and contrecoup injury, respectively). More prominent, however, are focal contusions of the anterior and inferior frontal and temporal lobes, occurring in the majority of cases of trauma (Adams, Graham, Murray, & Scott, 1982; Ommaya & Gennarelli, 1974). These regions are vulnerable to damage because the force of impact or rapid deceleration of the head causes movement of these parts of the brain against the jagged surfaces, prominences, and cavities of the inferior cranium. The back and forth movement tears brain tissue and small arteries along the surface of the brain.

The second type of primary brain injury is diffuse, widespread axonal damage caused by rotational force and stretching of nerve fibers (Pang, 1985). Diffuse axonal injury (DAI) is a common neuropathological find-

Table 1-1.   Types of injury to the brain as a result of a closed head injury.

Primary brain injury

Focal brain injury

Coup or impact injury

Contrecoup injury

Frontal lobes

Temporal lobes

Diffuse brain injury–Diffuse axonal injury

Secondary brain injury

Hematomas

Swelling

Edema

Increased intracranial pressure

Ischemia

Anoxia or hypoxia

ing in rapid acceleration-deceleration injuries such as motor vehicle accidents and is discovered visually only on microscopic examination (Adams et al., 1982). Animal studies have suggested that the length of coma and functional outcome are related to the severity of DAI (Gennarelli et al., 1982). In more severe cases of brain injury, additional white matter lesions tend to occur in the corpus callosum, the rostal brainstem, and the superior cerebellar peduncles (Strich, 1969).

Secondary brain injury is the result of pathologic processes set in action by the primary damage. These potential complications, as shown in Table 1-1, include hematomas or bleeding within the brain, brain swelling, edema, increased intracranial pressure, ischemia, and anoxia. More detailed descriptions of the neuropathology of trauma can be found in Adams, Graham, and Gennarelli (1985), Graham et al. (1987), and Pang (1985).

Therefore, the resulting damage to the brain after trauma is a complex permutation of these primary and secondary injuries (Pang, 1985). Because of the possibility of both multifocal and widespread damage, virtually every aspect of human thinking and behavior can be affected. Changes in sensory, motor, cognitive, linguistic, behavioral, social, and emotional functioning are found, with varying severity levels and differing degrees of interaction. This means that the changes stemming from a brain injury are multidimensional, complex, and variable.

Preinjury Functioning

A second major factor shown in Figure 1-1 that contributes to the heterogeneity of this population is the interaction of the injury and the person. As Sir Charles Symonds (1937) stated, "It is not only the kind of injury that matters, but the kind of head." Factors such as premorbid education, intelligence, personality, motivation, psychosocial functioning, and occupational status are potent factors in the outcome of brain injury (Brooks, McKinlay, Symington, Beattie, & Campsie, 1987; Gilchrist & Wilkinson, 1979; Rimel, Giordani, Barth, Boll, & Jane, 1981).

Social and Environmental Influences

As displayed in Figure 1-1, a third factor in the diversity of individual functioning and outcome after TBI includes social and environmental factors. Each individual's recovery is shaped by his or her unique familial, cultural, and social influences and by the physical environment. Family and cultural attitudes toward disability affect the expression of symptoms and outcomes in many ways. Certain families and cultures foster dependance for individuals with disabilities or feel a sense of shame or guilt. The willingness and ability of a family to provide support for an individual can determine the needed residential placement for many persons with brain injuries. Without a family capable and willing to provide assistance or advocate for services, some individuals experience less favorable outcomes.

Secondary Reaction to Injury

As displayed in Figure 1-1, another interwoven source of individual variation is an individual's reaction to an injury and the circumstances. Psychological resources and coping abilities of an individual affect outcome. Unfortunately, adaptive and coping capabilities may, themselves, be adversely affected by the injury or the postinjury environment.

Time and Recovery

A final factor contributing to the extraordinary range of individual variation in the consequences of brain injury has to do with chronicity, the time span from injury and events up to a given point in terms of rehabilitation and recovery. The expression of the injury varies depending on these factors. The needs of individuals 1 month after injury are much different from those at 6 months, which in turn might be different from those at 12 months. Where the individual is in the recovery process and what services have been provided to assist in recovery contribute to the heterogeneity of this population.

Frontal Lobe Dysfunction

Despite the variability of this population, there is one common factor; virtually all individuals with TBI sustain damage to the prefrontal cortex, the portion of the frontal lobes anterior to the primary and supplementary motor areas (Adams, Graham, Scott, Parker, & Doyle, 1980; Mattson & Levin, 1990). This presents several challenges to clinicians. One is that the functions of the prefrontal cortex have not been clearly delineated to this point. Second, the frontal lobes serve a complex role, exerting "executive" control of higher human behavior by regulating and integrating cognitive and behavioral functioning. These functions are vital aspects of human functioning, yet there are few guidelines for assessing and rehabilitating them.

The various functions of the prefrontal lobes include goal setting, initiation of goal-directed behavior, appraisal/evaluation of one's own performance, problem solving, organization of input, planning and sequencing of behavior, and inhibition of inappropriate behavior. The influence of executive dysfunction on rehabilitation and community reintegration has become increasingly clear (Grafman, Sirigu, Spector, & Hendler, 1993; Lezak, 1982, 1987b; Schwartz, Mayer, Fitzpatrick De Salme, & Montgomery, 1993; Varney & Menefee, 1993; Ylvisaker, 1992).

One aspect of frontal lobe dysfunction that poses a particular challenge for rehabilitation professionals is diminished self-awareness (Lam, McMahon, Priddy, & Gehred-Schultze, 1988; Prigatano, Altman, & O'Brien, 1990). Many individuals with frontal lobe damage have difficulty with realistic appraisal of their performance and abilities. Physical changes, such as limb weakness or dysarthria, are generally acknowledged and even cognitive changes may be inconsistently reported. Behavioral or psychosocial changes, on the other hand, tend to be underestimated by these individuals (Fordyce & Roueche, 1986; Prigatano et al., 1990). Insight regarding the ramifications of postinjury changes on their life goals and their families is often lacking. Because of this, individuals with brain injury may have difficulty understanding the need for rehabilitation and accepting the feedback of others when it differs from their own perception. An individual may lack motivation to use compensatory strategies or to maintain gains made from therapy. An individual's level of participation, cooperation, and appreciation is often sorely disappointing to a clinician.

Another aspect of executive functioning that seriously affects rehabilitation is the regulation of drive or output (Lezak, 1982; Ylvisaker, 1992). Individuals with severely reduced drive or initiation may not be able to generate the mental effort required to become fully and actively engaged in their own treatment. They may fail to initiate the use of the skills and strategies acquired through rehabilitation. On the other hand, individuals with severe disinhibition may fail to use learned skills and strategies because of impulsivity and, therefore, always be a risk in terms of safety despite adequate functional skills (Ylvisaker, 1992).

Despite current limitations in conceptualizing the multiple roles of the frontal lobes, progress has been made in the last several years (see Hart & Jacobs, 1993; Shallice & Burgess, 1991). These developments will be covered in Chapters 2 and 3.

Psychiatric Disturbances

Another difficult aspect of brain injury for clinicians to manage are the psychiatric disturbances. Most commonly encountered are challenging behaviors, such as aggression and inappropriate sexual behavior. Working with individuals with these symptoms is often frustrating and demanding and may lead to embarrassment and even fear. The argumentative nature, impatience, and irritability of some individuals with brain injuries result in stress and anger for both clinicians and families (Cavallo, Kay, & Ezrachi, 1992; Prigatano, 1989). Few clinicians, however, receive training in managing these behaviors, and few rehabilitation programs are organized to address these issues in a structured and systematic manner (Wood, 1987).

Other psychiatric concerns include depression, immature behavior, anxiety, mania, obsessive compulsive behavior, and paranoid or delusional behavior. The origin of these disturbances is generally multifaceted, being affected by premorbid characteristics, the injury, and the environment.

Financial and Ethical Considerations

Unfortunately, to this point, access to appropriate rehabilitation is all too often determined by a person's financial resources. Clinicians may face conflicts between the desire to meet an individual's needs and the lack of funding. Even for those clients with funding, the influence of cost containment forces on rehabilitation has resulted in shorter lengths of stay, decreased reimbursement, and more difficulty in obtaining and keeping coverage for services.

An additional issue has to do with allegations of fraud and unethical practices within for-profit brain injury programs. Unfortunately, some consumers and lay persons have developed mistrust of the whole field because of alleged billing fraud, unethical clinical services, and unethical marketing practices of these corporations (Committee on Government Operations, 1992). Clinicians working in these settings may find themselves faced with ethical dilemmas concerning the good of the individual versus the good of the company and with consumers skeptical of their professional ethics and efforts.

The Role of the Speech-Language Pathologist

Due to the complex neuropathology of TBI and resulting changes in functioning, communication disorders encountered by speech-language pathologists are complex and varied. Swallowing disorders, motor speech and voice disorders, aphasia, and cognitive-communicative disorders may appear alone or in combination. Cognitive-communicative disorders are defined as alterations in communication due to deficits in a variety of linguistic and nonlinguistic cognitive processes (American Speech-Language-Hearing Association [ASHA], 1991). These cognitive processes include executive functioning, attention, information processing, memory, visuospatial perception, reasoning/problem solving, and psychosocial behavior. Examples of resulting communication deficits include difficulty attending to and understanding complex commands, difficulty retaining information from a story, inability to organize spoken expression so that it is coherent and to the point, and difficulty selecting appropriate topics of conversation.

Frequently, the four types of communication disorders coexist, especially immediately after injury in the acute stage of recovery. The prominence and/or relative significance of each (and, therefore, treatment focus), however, may vary with the stage of recovery and pattern of injury. Immediately after injury, in an acute hospital or a subacute rehabilitation setting, when the individual is in coma, intubated, or emerging from coma, intervention is focused on swallowing, orientation, facilitation of basic information processing, and reestablishment of a means of basic communication. Once an individual is generally oriented, treatment concentrates on rebuilding motor control for speech, if necessary, and component linguistic and nonlinguistic cognitive abilities, such as auditory comprehension, attention and memory (Adamovich, Henderson, & Auerbach, 1985; Sohlberg & Mateer, 1989b; Ylvisaker, 1985).

When a client begins to demonstrate purposeful and generally appropriate behavior, the emphasis of treatment should shift more and more to the reestablishment (or establishment) of functional life skills (Szekeres, Ylvisaker, & Holland, 1985). The term *functional* as used here means pertaining to an individual's everyday, real-world activities. Therefore, *functional communication* means those communication skills necessary for an individual to communicate adequately and appropriately in his or her own daily living, work, social, academic, leisure, or community activities. Functional communication skills include describing symptoms of illness to a physician, carrying on a conversation with a loved one, following directions in physical therapy, calling a taxi, or taking notes in class. The term functional communication is used in a broad sense, encompassing social communication or interpersonal communication and the use of intrapersonal language for learning and behavioral control.

Although some individuals continue to demonstrate motor speech disorder or aphasia at the postacute stage, virtually all moderately to severely injured individuals experience problems in functional communication because of changes in their cognitive-communicative abilities (Hartley & Jensen, 1991; Liles, Coelho, Duffy, & Zalagens, 1989; Marsh & Knight,

1991; Mentis & Prutting, 1987; Milton, Prutting, & Binder, 1984; Prigatano, Roueche, & Fordyce, 1986). It is critical for clinicians to address functional communication needs to achieve success in rehabilitation at the postacute level. This need is particularly apparent when one examines the literature on long-term outcomes, understands the limitations of previous approaches to communication disorders, and recognizes the need for cost-effective and individually defined approaches to rehabilitation.

Rationale for a Functional Perspective

Addressing Major Barriers to Successful Outcomes

Both research and clinical literature now provide insight into the long-term outcomes of brain injury and barriers to successful rehabilitation and community reintegration. These are listed in Table 1–2. Ineffective interpersonal skills are now felt to be the major cause of poor long-term outcomes (Ben-Yishay, Silver, Piasetsky, & Rattok, 1987; Lezak, 1987b; Malkmus, 1989; Prigatano, 1987). Problems in interpersonal situations affect the ability to form and maintain meaningful and satisfying personal relationships in every aspect of life. Oddy and his colleagues (Oddy, 1984; Oddy & Humphrey, 1980; Oddy et al., 1978) found social isolation to be the most devastating long-term consequence of brain injury. Contributing factors included confusion (forgetfulness) and verbal expansiveness (brash, outspoken, verbally aggressive). Families report more distress in coping with the disturbed interpersonal interactions of their loved one than with physical changes (McKinlay, Brooks, Bond, Martinage, & Marshall, 1981).

Problems in functional communication have been found to be significant factors in failure to return to work and to maintain employment (Ben-Yishay, Silver et al., 1987; Brooks et al., 1987; Jacobs, 1988). Even the quality of residential care and rehabilitation is influenced by interpersonal behavior (Wood, 1987). This body of research points out the crucial need for rehabilitation to specifically build functional communication abilities.

A second, but related, major barrier to successful outcomes, as shown in Table 1–2, is frontal lobe dysfunction. Changes in frontal lobe function-

Table 1–2.   Barriers to successful outcomes.

Ineffective interpersonal skills

Frontal lobe dysfunction

   Decreased self-awareness

   Decreased regulation

Challenges to learning and applying new information

ing are felt to be a major cause of these psychosocial changes. As stated earlier, reduced awareness of deficits and impaired regulation of goal-directed behavior are common areas of concern with frontal lobe dysfunction. Because of these changes, individuals with brain injury often refuse to cooperate or make little effort, unless they perceive that therapeutic tasks have significance to their personal goals and desires (Ylvisaker, 1992). Therefore, it is paramount with this population that intervention have *face validity*—that is, that chosen tasks, methods, and materials readily convey the relevance of intervention to an individual's everyday functional needs.

A third known barrier to successful outcomes in rehabilitation is the network of learning problems associated with brain injury. Individuals with brain injury frequently have problems in acquiring new learning and with generalizing and transferring any learning that does occur (Parente & DiCesare, 1991). Functional skills training, however, capitalizes on an intact learning ability—procedural memory, or the ability to learn a task consisting of a series of actions by actually performing it a number of times. Classroom lectures, discussions, and paper-and-pencil tasks are often not as effective teaching methods as intervention in real-life events for this population. In addition, by training behaviors that are of functional significance in a variety of natural settings and with a variety of interaction partners, generalization is more likely to occur (Kearns, 1989). Teaching the specific skills that are needed in identified daily living or work activities facilitates the transfer of learning (Parente & DiCesare, 1991).

Limitations of Previous Approaches

Another impetus for assuming a more functional approach is a paradigmatic shift that has occurred over the past two decades, first in social sciences and then in clinical domains. The older positivist paradigm called for quantitative methods of data collection under highly controlled conditions and statistical analysis (Butler, 1990). The traditional methods of assessment and treatment of neurologic communication disorders were the product of this paradigm. As shown in Table 1–3, the focus in this approach was on isolated linguistic skills, with great efforts made to avoid the "confounding" effects of context or nonlinguistic factors. These methods were developed to precisely and reliably measure the presence and severity of deficits in component processes, such as comprehension of spoken language, in discrete units (words, phrases, sentences). Administration was always conducted in structured, clinical settings. Performance was judged as to accuracy and perhaps latency of response. Deficits were identified and treatment goals were designed to reduce the deficiencies in component processes.

A gradual paradigmatic shift occurred first in philosophy, sociology, linguistics, and anthropology, and later in the more clinically related fields

Table 1-3.   Comparison of traditional and functional approaches to assessment and treatment.

	Traditional	Functional
Focus	Linguistic skills	Communication, including cognitive and psychosocial factors
Units of measure	Component processes Words, grammatical structures	Connected speech, discourse, social interaction
Setting	Clinic, structured activities	Real world, everyday tasks
Scoring	Accuracy, time	Effectiveness, appropriateness
Purpose	Diagnose aphasia presence, type, severity Measure impairments	Use of residual strengths Compensatory strategies Determine disability

of education, speech-language pathology, and psychology. The postpositivist paradigm places increased emphasis on qualitative research methods that permit the study of behaviors and relationships in natural settings and activities (Butler, 1990; Garrison, 1986). This paradigmatic shift within linguistics resulted in the field of pragmatics, or the study of language in natural contexts, and in discourse analysis. These developments, in turn, impacted the field of speech-language pathology by broadening our view of communication and providing a theoretical basis for understanding language and language disruption in natural contexts. From anthropology comes ethnographic methods for describing and analyzing language as it occurs within day-to-day activities (Ripich & Spinelli, 1985).

When viewed from a postpositivist perspective, the *ecological* or *social validity* of traditional approaches to neurogenic communication disorders became questionable. Ecological or social validity concerns the generalizibililty of evaluation or treatment results under controlled situations to natural environments (Tupper & Cicerone, 1990). Research and clinical experience have demonstrated that the results of traditional aphasia batteries do not provide a complete picture of communication abilities in real life; these tests tend to underestimate the functional communication of adults with aphasia and overestimate the functional communication of individuals with traumatic brain injury or right hemisphere damage (Holland, 1982; Milton et al., 1984). In addition, these traditional assessment tools do not lead readily to socially valid treatment goals and may be insensitive to functional improvements that may occur from treatment (Aten, Caligiuri, & Holland, 1982; Sarno & Levita, 1979).

In contrast to traditional methods, a postpositivist or functional approach to assessing neurologic communication disorders, as outlined in

Table 1–3, considers psychosocial and cognitive as well as linguistic factors in the performance of everyday communication activities. Discourse is the basic unit of measurement, and assessment occurs in the real world as well as clinical settings. Adequacy, effectiveness, and appropriateness form the bases for judging performance. Evaluation assesses not only deficits, but also preserved abilities and self-generated compensatory strategies. Treatment occurs within natural settings using everyday tasks to capitalize on strengths as well as address areas of weakness.

Accountability for Functional Outcomes

Rehabilitation has been influenced by this paradigmatic shift as well, resulting in a reframing of its purpose. Unfortunately, treatment cannot completely cure or totally restore function for the majority of severely injured individuals. Research has shown that, in most cases, the underlying impairments (e.g., memory deficits, poor initiation) will be long-term if not lifelong issues. Rehabilitation must teach a person how to live with these impairments. In other words, treatment at some point must seek not just to diminish the impairments but to lessen the disability, or functional limitations, caused by the impairments. Services must be organized by first identifying the targeted discharge disposition of an individual and then, based on this information, developing services to make the discharge option a reality (Whitman, 1991).

Consumers and third-party payers are looking more closely at functional outcomes of rehabilitation. With the proliferation of facilities, high cost of services, and increased knowledge and expectations for brain injury rehabilitation, consumers and funding sources, alike, are questioning how the services delivered will impact real-life abilities (functional skills and quality of life) and affect bottom-line costs (length of treatment, level of long-term care required). Everyone involved wants to achieve the best functional outcomes in the shortest amount of time. Insurance case managers and other funding representatives are insisting on this for cost-containment.

In an effort to address these quality assurance and accountability concerns, clinicians are being asked to produce documentation about functional abilities and projected functional outcomes—in other words, to be accountable for results beyond the clincal setting. Medicare requires clinicians to develop functional goals. Accrediting bodies such as the Commission for the Accreditation of Rehabilitation Facilities (CARF) require use of functional measures of outcome to determine treatment effectiveness. Federal agencies, such as the National Institute on Disability and Rehabilitation Research and the newly formed National Center for Medical Rehabilitation Research, have placed the development of better measures of functional outcomes as a major funding priority. The

American Speech-Language-Hearing Association has recognized the importance of functional measures by developing a comprehensive scale of functional communication (Frattali, personal communication, June 14, 1993).

Influence of the Disability Movement

Another impetus for the development of more functional or ecologically valid approaches to rehabilitation has been the disability and independent living movement. Consumers want and are demanding a more active part in determining their treatment and its outcome in all aspects of health care and human service. They have forced providers to rethink their model of service delivery.

As stated by Condeluci (1992), human services are often driven by the medical model. In this model, the professional is seen as the expert who takes charge of treatment, and the "patient" is expected to comply. The focus is on identifying the problems within the person and treating the isolated deficits. Patients are segregated with others considered just like themselves.

The alternative model, Condeluci purposes, is an "interdependent model." The individual is empowered to make informed choices, and treatment is focused on the individual's capacities and the development of interrelationships and interconnections. The perceived problem is not within a person, but within society, in terms of the provision of the necessary supports and structures for a person to fully participate in the community. This, Condeluci argues, is the model under which the community reintegration phase of rehabilitation must operate.

The concepts of normalization and social role valorization are the philosophical underpinnings for service delivery in this model. As outlined by Wolfensberger (1983) and Condeluci and Gretz-Lasky (1987), persons with disabilities have the right to live as normal a life as possible, with the dignity to risk, make decisions concerning their lives, and pursue normal relationships. Service providers must promote the value of the social role of individuals with disabilities by employing activities and treatment methods that are culturally normative and age-appropriate. The professional is seen as a partner in the process of expanding the options and opportunities for an individual within the community. Responsibility for educating the community about brain injury and identifying community supports is also an integral role of the professional in this new perspective.

Service delivery systems have been heavily influenced by this consumer-driven model. CARF standards require that rehabilitation programs make the individual served and his or her family a vital part of the rehabilitation team and involved in every aspect of decision-making. The passage of the Americans with Disabilities Act (ADA), a product of this movement, has helped to create more options for individuals with disabilities and has raised society's consciousness about the rights of these individuals, as well as the need to make "reasonable accommodations."

In summary, this section has presented a rationale for a functional approach to cognitive-communicative abilities after TBI:

1. Ineffective social communication is a major barrier to successful community reintegration.

2. Individuals with brain injury need to believe that treatment has relevance to their lives.

3. Functional skill training in functional settings helps to overcome challenges faced by persons with TBI in the acquisition of new learning, generalization, and transfer of skills.

4. Individuals with TBI have a right to rehabilitation with individually defined goals that result in socially meaningful outcomes.

5. Improved functional abilities are the end goal of all rehabilitation.

6. Theoretical and clinical guidelines now exist for a more functional approach to cognitive-communication disorders.

Defining a Functional Approach

This chapter has hopefully created an understanding of the complexities and needs of individuals who have sustained brain injuries and their families, especially at the later stages of recovery when the focus is achievement of the highest level of community reintegration possible. As Malkmus (1989) stated, this postacute stage of rehabilitation "bridges the gap between the medical setting and the social world" (p. 53) to achieve the highest level of functioning in living, social, work, and academic activities. A number of reasons have been presented for employing a functional approach to cognitive-communication behaviors with this population—to focus on functional skills and functional outcomes. In summarizing the key ideas and concepts and to translate them into the clinical process, a definition of a functional approach is now more fully articulated.

A functional approach to cognitive-communication disorders can be viewed from three angles. As outlined in Table 1–4, a functional approach can be viewed as a philosophy of rehabilitation, an intervention strategy, and a guide to the content of intervention (Valletutti & Dummett, 1992). As a philosophy, it embraces the value of functional life roles and responsibilities. This means that the mission of clinicians is to assist individuals in the performance of social roles and to empower individuals served to make informed choices. A functional approach promotes a normalizing, interdependent model of service to rehabilitation, building independence

Table 1-4.   Defining a functional approach.

A *philosophy of rehabilitation*

    Social role valorization

    Empowerment

    Normalization

    Interdependent model of service

    Consumer-driven

    Ecological validity

An *intervention strategy*

    Top-down process

    Outcome-oriented

    Holistic

    Natural environments

A *guide to content*

    Normal adult social roles

    Personally meaningful tasks and content

    Functional life skills

---

when appropriate and building use of natural and community supports when interdependence is more appropriate. It optimizes the active participation of the individual and the individualization of treatment, tailoring the program to an individual's unique set of preferences, strengths, needs, and values (Malkmus, 1989). It is an ecologically valid approach that emphasizes development of social competence or effectiveness in meeting the standards and social demands of an individual's own cultural and social environment (Malkmus, 1989).

As an intervention strategy (see Table 1-4), a functional approach employs a top-down path; that is, the desired outcomes, based on typical adult roles and activities, are identified first and competencies needed for those outcomes are then the target for intervention (Whitman, 1991). This implies that a holistic approach will be used that considers an individual's social, cultural, and physical environment in both evaluation and intervention procedures. It also means that functional skills must be taught functionally through actual experiences in natural contexts or settings whenever possible (Valletutti & Dummett, 1992).

Employing a functional approach shapes the content of intervention in a number of ways. Communication skills that are relevant to the daily behavior expected of adults are given primary concern. All content must be evaluated in relationship to its relevance to the development of responsible, effective, and successful personal and social adaptation. Priorities must be given to the development of competencies within the specific contexts relevant to an individual.

Summary

This chapter has emphasized that individuals with brain injuries have complex, multiple changes in their functional or social communication abilities and that these changes often are responsible for the difficulties experienced in long-term community reintegration. A functional approach is necessary to reestablish competency in social communication and efficiently achieve functional outcomes in the areas of daily living, leisure, social, consumer, academic, and work activities.

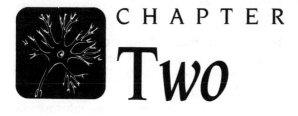

C H A P T E R

Two

A Model for Understanding Social Communication Following Brain Injury

Armed with a rationale and philosophy for a functional approach, we now must search for a road map to get us to our destination. We still must face the questions: What is functional communication? How do you determine communicative, or social, competence? As stated in Chapter 1, because of additional intrapersonal and interpersonal influences on communication in natural settings, communicative competence goes beyond linguistic competence. Functional communication consists of a complex repertoire of dynamic social behaviors that require the integration of one's knowledge of the world with cognitive, social, behavioral, psychological, and linguistic processes. Human behaviors, however, do not occur in a vacuum; the environment in which functions occur is a major determinant of communication behavior.

When searching the literature, it is evident that social communication is the concern of many different fields of study, each viewing it from a slightly different angle. Considering the multidimensional nature of everyday communication, this is not surprising. This means, however, that clinicians interested in communicative competence need a solid theoretical foundation derived from the perspectives of various fields. Table 2–1 lists a number of fields of study that have contributed to our understanding of social communication, with selected topics and references. Information from all of these areas has been integrated into a model of social communication that is outlined and related to communication competence after brain injury in this chapter.

Overview of a Model of Social Communication

Communication competence is defined by Larson, Backlund, Redmond, and Barbour (1978) as "the ability to demonstrate knowledge of the communication behavior socially appropriate to a given situation" (p. 21). Spitzberg (1983) and Spitzberg and Hurt (1987) suggest that communication competency should be viewed as interpersonal relational competency and judged on a continuum of effectiveness and appropriateness.

Due to its complexity, there is no clear consensus on the various components of communication competence. Five elements were considered by Spitzberg and Hurt (1987) to be relevant to interpersonal competence: motivation for communication, knowledge of communication, skill in communicating, sensitivity to the context, and achievement of desired outcomes. This concept of communication, however, does not take into consideration information processing or neuropsychological aspects of comprehending and producing everyday language.

The model of social communication used in this book is shown in Figure 2–1. The model is both linear and circular to denote the dynamic, ongoing, and cyclical nature of communicative interactions. That is, natural communication does not occur in a preset, rigid order, but evolves over time as the communicative behavior of one person interfaces with that of another person within an ongoing situation. The cyclical pattern also denotes the cybernetic nature of human behavior. An individual receives and decodes sensory input from the environment, generates an appropriate behavioral response, and refines and modifies the behavior, based internal monitoring of the behavior, and its effect on the environment.

The arrows in the model also indicate that the processes of social communication do not occur in a strictly serial or unidirectional manner, but are interactive, with both top-down as well as bottom-up processing. That is, comprehension can be viewed as starting at the "bottom" level of processing, by attending to, perceiving, and comprehending linguistic in-

Table 2-1. Fields of study relevant to social communication.

Areas	Topics	Selected References
Behavioral and Clinical Psychology	Social skills/competence Behavioral analysis Assertiveness Social problem solving	Arkowitz, 1981; Bellack, 1983; Conger, Moisan-Thomas, & Conger, 1989; Curran & Monti, 1982; Goldstein, Sprafkin, Gershaw, & Klein, 1980; Jacobs, 1993
Cognitive Psychology	Schemata and scripts Memory processes Information processing	Bower, Black, & Turner, 1979; Kellermann, Broetzmann, Lim, & Kitao, 1989; Schank & Abelson, 1977; Tulving, 1985
Linguistics and Sociolinguistics	Pragmatics Discourse processes Discourse grammar Accommodation theory Ethnography	Grice, 1975; Hamilton, 1991; Labov, 1972; Searle, 1969; Stein & Glenn, 1979; van Dijk, 1977; Winograd, 1977
Speech-Language Pathology and Neurolinguistics	Pragmatic assessment Discourse processes Functional communication Social skills/conversation	Beukelman, Yorkston, & Lossing, 1984; Davis & Wilcox, 1985; Joanette & Brownell, 1990; Mentis & Prutting, 1987, 1991; Milton, 1988, Prutting & Kirchner, 1983; 1987; Sarno, 1984a; Wiig, 1982a; Ylvisaker, 1992
Speech Communication	Communicative competence Relationship development	Applegate & Leichty, 1984; Cooley & Roach, 1984; Spitzberg & Hurt, 1987
Neuropsychology	Cognitive, executive, and neurobehavioral influences on communication	Alexander, Benson, & Stuss, 1989; Hart & Jacobs, 1993; Levin, Eisenberg, & Benton, 1991; Lezak, 1982, 1987b, 1989; Prigatano, 1987; Wood, 1987
Education	Life skills training Language/Second language	Lundsteen, 1979; Valletutti & Dummett, 1992

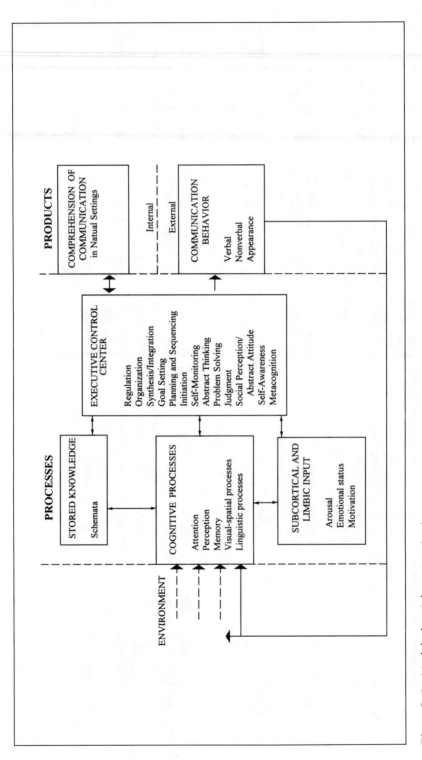

Figure 2–1. Model of social communication.

put. Simultaneously, however, "top" level processes (from the executive control center in the model) exert influence on comprehension, such as when a student intentionally increases attention when a teacher says, "In order to pass the exam, you need to . . .".

The model of social communication presented in Figure 2–1 can be subdivided in several ways. It depicts that understanding of social communication and performance of social skills are products of the interaction of our environment with our internal states, knowledge, and processing capabilities. Viewed from another angle, it illustrates that interpersonal behavior is a result of interaction between an individual's environment and an individual's internal functioning. It also denotes that social communicative performance can be viewed separately from social knowledge and comprehension. In other words, a person may have superior knowledge of appropriate behavior and understand communication, but not be a skilled performer of social communication.

The model outlines the processes involved both in comprehension of social communication and in production of communicative behavior. Although encoding and decoding occur simultaneously in natural settings, each will be traced separately through the model to demonstrate the steps involved. Understanding social communication requires rapid processing of continuous verbal and nonverbal input from the environment, possibly from multiple speakers, and retention of this input, as well as retention of what has occurred earlier in the interaction and in the environment. Processing capacity must be divided between continuously encoding the contextual data while maintaining information long enough to integrate this external input with internal world knowledge and value, motivational, and belief systems. Strategies for organizing the input, retrieving relevant knowledge, making inferences about relationships, goals, and meaning, making critical judgments about the message or participant, anticipating what will be said or done next based on prior knowledge, and monitoring one's comprehension are applied by a control center for information processing, here called the executive control center, a function of the prefrontal cortex.

The model in Figure 2–1 also conceptualizes the multiple aspects of the generation of social communication. Social behavior is initiated and maintained by an overall goal formed by the executive control center. An overall plan of what needs to occur is based on an individual's perception and understanding of relevant dimensions of a communicative situation (Trower, Bryant, & Argyle, 1978). To implement this plan, the executive control center must integrate these perceptions with stored knowledge and with input regarding current emotional/motivational status to determine possible courses of action to accomplish the desired goal. The executive control center then considers the effectiveness and appropriateness of each possibility before deciding the best course of action. The plan is then implemented through activation of a particular schema from stored knowledge and specific linguistic and motor responses. The control center continuously monitors and evaluates the chosen social behavior, making adjustments and adaptations based on internal and environmental feedback.

As described in Chapter 1, changes in communication are a major concern after traumatic brain injury (TBI), because of the tremendous impact on information processing, interpersonal skills, social problem solving, and regulation of behavior. Individuals often fail to select the right time and place for interactions, to adapt their communication style to the demands of the social or physical context, to fully comprehend conversation in natural settings, to express their thoughts and ideas in a clear and concise manner, or to follow social/cultural rules of discourse. Next, this chapter clarifies the components of social communication diagramed in Figure 2–1 and considers the nature of communication deficits following brain injury.

The Environment: Contexts of Communication

Bickhard (1987) defines natural language as a complex goal-directed, interactional behavioral system requiring sensitivity to the environment to be successful in reaching its goal. As Prutting (1982) states, "There is no way to interpret social competence unless communicative behavior and context are treated simultaneously" (p. 132). The ability to monitor the context of communication is a prerequisite for appropriate, effective, and successful communicative interactions with others (Prutting, 1982).

Context "is the interrelated conditions in which something exists or occurs" (Prutting, 1982, p. 125). Although both external and internal contexts exist, "environment," or context, is used here to mean the situations or conditions in which communication occurs external to a person. Four major aspects of context, as described by Davis and Wilcox (1985), Levinson (1983), Prutting (1982), Winograd (1977), are outlined in Table 2–2. These include the social and cognitive context, the physical context, the linguistic context, and the nonverbal context.

Social and Cognitive Context

One of the primary aspects of context is that communication functions in a social setting. As a socially interactive process, communication requires cooperation and participation in alternating roles as listener and speaker. In addition, social factors such as relative social status, authority, age, and relationship (level of familiarity/intimacy) of the participants must be considered when formulating an appropriate speech style and register,

Table 2-2.   The contexts of communication.

Social and Cognitive Context
  Roles as speaker and as receiver
  Relative social status—perceived status, power, authority, age
  Relationship—level of intimacy
  Cultural background of participants
  Emotional and cognitive status of partner
  Shared knowledge of participants
  Individual goals and intentions
  Overall purpose of interaction

Physical Context
  Physical surroundings
  Time
  Location of participants and objects
  Number of individuals present

Linguistic Context

Nonverbal Context

topics, and degree of politeness and directness. For example, speakers alter the tone of voice, degree of politeness, degree of self-disclosure, topic of conversation, and formality of conversation depending on whether they are speaking to a spouse or a supervisor.

The cultural background of the participants is another aspect of the social context of communication. Our values, beliefs, stereotypes, and prejudices are shaped by our culture and influence how we interact with others, especially persons from a different cultural or ethnic background.

Each participant is expected to be sensitive to the cognitive and emotional status of the communication partner. This sensitivity requires individuals to be aware that other persons have beliefs and perceptions that guide their behavior and that those beliefs and perceptions may be different from those of themselves. In developmental psychology this is known as the "theory of mind" (Ashington, Harris, & Olson, 1988). The ability to infer mental states and use the inferences to predict behavior is the origin of feelings of empathy. This ability begins to emerge at the age of 4 to 5 and becomes more fully operational by age 7 to 8 (Wimmer & Perner, 1983).

The emotional status of the listener may impact the communicative competence of the speaker. Bellack (1983) notes that the degree of social skill and effectiveness of an individual is affected by the responsiveness, cooperation, and affective state (mood, anxiety) of a communication partner. In other words, a person may have difficulty communicating effectively to a hostile, uncooperative, or nonresponsive individual.

Speakers are expected to modify their verbal output based on knowledge of a listener's ability to process. In other words, speakers assess their listeners in terms of what is known, what is in active memory, what is the focus of attention, and what is shared knowledge. This ability to take the listener's perspective and adapt a message to the needs of the listener is called "role-taking ability," or "perspective-taking ability" (McTear & Conti-Ramsden, 1992). Speakers will vary the specificity of reference to objects and events and the amount of information they give, based on a speaker's assumption of the listener's knowledge and ability to understand the message. For example, a speaker will provide fewer details on how to get to his or her house when the listener is familiar with the neighborhood than when the listener is new to the area.

The goals and intentions of the participants as well as the overriding purpose of the social interaction are other facets of the social context. For example, a television commercial for dog food or a telephone sales pitch for water softeners is very different from standard conversation. A wedding is much more highly ritualized than a party situation. You may respond differently to a friend asking for a favor for the fifth time as opposed to the same friend interested in finding out if he or she can do something for you.

Physical Context

The physical and temporal setting of the communication is a second major contextual consideration. We operate with certain guidelines for conversation in specific environments—for example, conversation on the tennis court as opposed to conversation at church. We choose a time and place to speak that is deemed by our culture to be appropriate, at a point that will increase the likelihood of a receptive response. Proximity of objects and persons influences our choice of terms as well. If items referred to are in view, they do not have to be as precisely described. The number of observers or partners is an additional factor, as most speakers are less nervous in one-on-one communication than in a group.

In certain instances, the physical context influences the channels of communication available; telephone communication relies more heavily on explicit, clear communication than does face-to-face interaction, with environmental and nonverbal cues being accessible (Roth & Spekman, 1984).

Linguistic and Nonverbal Context

Prior and co-occurring verbal and nonverbal behavior are additional contextual variables that constrain communication behavior. Verbal behavior is somewhat elusive, because of the imprecise nature of expressing feelings, desires, beliefs, and motivations through language (Prutting, 1982). Non-verbal communication is even more elusive and subtle, with much of it conducted at the unconscious level of awareness (Bateson, 1972).

Sensitivity to Context Following Brain Injury

One of the major characteristics of communication after TBI is difficulty in the use of situationally appropriate communication behavior. Many individuals act as though they are not aware of the social and cultural rules that dictate the selection of appropriate behavior for the environment. For example, Wayne would continue to talk regardless of multiple nonverbal cues that a staff member was busy or wanted him to leave. One day a secretary, desperate to end a conversation with him, headed for the rest room. He would have followed her right into the ladies' room, talking away, had she not physically stopped him at the door.

This lack of adaptation to the communication environment has multiple possible causes, involving each component of the model in Figure 2–1. It can be caused by problems in cognitive processes, a lack of knowledge of the social rules, poor motivation to consider the environment, inadequate social performance skills, or poor executive control over the use and integration of each of these components. Each of these components will be examined separately.

Subcortical and Limbic Input:
Arousal, Motivational, and Mood Status

The brain's subcortical regions and limbic system influence our processing and behavior in a number of ways. The reticular activating system (RAS) (Moruzzi & Magoun, 1949) of the brain stem has a major influence on the general arousal or activation level of the brain and activation of the autonomic nervous system (Kløve, 1987). As Kløve points out, the state of arousal can be conceived as a continuum, ranging from deep sleep or coma at one end to a hyperaroused state of panic at the other. Adequate and efficient cognitive processing and emotional control require a certain arousal level; underactivation or overactivation is detrimental to human functioning.

The RAS and, thus, our arousal state is influenced by the amount of external stimulation (sensory input), internal stimulation (sleep-wake cycles, normal body rhythms, cardiopulmonary functioning, and metabolic or nutritional status), and stress (alcohol, drugs, anxiety, and fatigue). When the arousal state is diminished, decrements in functioning can be noted in the other components of the model, most directly attentional processes, emotional-mood status, and motivation.

Our mood or emotional status can affect our processing in many ways, such as when increased communicative anxiety during a presentation causes us to forget parts of a prepared speech. On the other hand, depression can cause a person to avoid social interaction or to perform social skills in a less competent manner. Our emotional status is related to arousal, in that feelings generally have an intensity dimension (Prigatano, 1987). The limbic system, primarily the hypothalamus and amygdaloid complex (anterior and mesial temporal lobe), is believed to exert a major influence on our emotional-mood status (Pribram, 1971). Closely tied to this are the metabolic and endocrine regulatory functions of the limbic-subcortical systems that are associated with internal biological drive states. These drives, such as for sexual, affection, and hunger satisfaction, influence our level of arousal and our motivation for interaction. For most individuals, topics and interactions that tap into emotional needs, areas of interest, or basic needs are more likely to increase attention to and motivation for interaction.

Motivation is defined by Prigatano (1987) as "the complex feeling states that parallel hierarchical goal-seeking behavior" (p. 357). Motivation is shaped by many factors, including early life experiences and the belief and value system instilled by one's culture. Motivational forces exert influence over arousal/attentional processes and thereby affect social interaction by dampening or stimulating our efforts at processing or formulating appropriate responses. Regions of the brain believed to be important for motivation include the basal ganglia and its connections to the limbic system, particularly the hypothalamus (Pribram, 1971; Prigatano, 1987).

Arousal, Mood, and Motivation Following Brain Injury

The influence of subcortical and limbic input on every other component in the social communication model is of particular concern following TBI. Diffuse axonal injury, common with a closed head injury, typically affects the pathways connecting the subcortical and limbic structures with each other and with the prefrontal regions (Graham et al., 1987). Particularly sensitive to axonal damage is the reticular activating system, because of its multiple projections. Decrements in arousal are frequently reported after TBI, which, in turn, result in decreased orienting responses to stimulation and decreased cortical activation necessary for efficient information processing and behavioral control.

Changes in emotional and motivational responses, over and above those attributable to decreased arousal, are also common after TBI. This is not too surprising, considering the likelihood of damage to the anterior and mesial temporal lobe (part of the limbic system) and to the basal ganglia in closed head injury (Graham, Adams, & Doyle, 1978; Graham, et al., 1987). Emotional and motivational changes attributable to the actual damage to the brain include irritability, poor frustration tolerance, increased anger or rage, lability, uncontrollable laughter, uncooperativeness, paranoia, impulsivity, and adynamia (lack of drive).

Anxiety, depression, and diminished self-esteem have all been reported to be relatively frequent secondary reactions to TBI, especially 6 to 12 months postinjury (Levin, Grossman, Rose, & Teasdale, 1979; MacNiven & Finlayson, 1993; Newton & Johnson, 1985). Emotional distress and depression have been found to exacerbate cognitive impairments, with devastating negative consequences in social functioning (Lezak, 1987b; MacNiven & Finlayson, 1993; Sbordone, 1991).

Schemata: Stored Knowledge

Over the last decade, greater understanding has been gained regarding human memory systems and the vital role of our files of stored knowledge in both comprehending and producing natural communication (Frederiksen, Bracewell, Breuleux, & Renaud, 1990). As stated by Kellermann, Broetzmann, Lim, and Kitao (1989), conversation involves the interfacing of cognitive processes and prior knowledge. Just focusing on the overt behaviors involved in communication fails to account for how our knowledge guides and directs our conversation.

Real world knowledge has been hypothesized to be stored in two systems—episodic and semantic memory (Tulving, 1985). Episodic memory is defined as the acquisition and storage of personally experienced events and their temporal relationships. Examples include an individual's ability to recall a particular vacation in childhood or high school graduation night. In contrast, semantic memory is built up over time and consists of more abstract, general knowledge of the internal and external world. This knowledge is hypothesized to be stored in organized cognitive structures called *schemas* or *schemata* (Frederiksen et al., 1990; Graesser, 1981; van Dijk, 1977; Winograd, 1977).

Schemata are memory structures consisting of interrelated types of information that are formed through experience. They have been described as "concepts, beliefs, expectations, processes—virtually everything from past experiences that are used in making sense of things and actions" (McNeil, 1992, p. 19).

As displayed in Table 2–3, there are many types of schemata. The simplest type includes ordinary objects and *concepts* linked together in semantic networks. For example, the word "corn" would be stored with related concepts or information, such as yellow, vegetable, husk, cob, kernels, food for people and pigs, grown on a farm, popcorn, Indian corn, and so on. This type of semantic memory is thought to be formed and stored primarily in the temporal and parietal lobes (Goldman-Rakic, 1993).

Table 2-3. Types of stored knowledge or schemata.

Concepts

Scripts

Scenes or Appositions

Social Situational Rules for Interactions

Social Conventions for Politeness and Cooperation

Discourse Grammars or Structures

Another hypothesized type of schema is called *script*, or situation-specific action sequence. Scripts are knowledge structures of familiar, stereotypical situations such as going to the doctor, eating at a fast food restaurant, and having a birthday party (Bower, Black, & Turner, 1979; Schank, 1982; Schank & Abelson, 1977). Related concepts and series of events are stored in the script for a particular situation or episode (Benoit & Follert, 1986). An example of a script is outlined in Table 2-4.

An alternative view of the organization of action sequences employ *"appositions"* (Benoit & Follert, 1986), *scenes*, or memory organization packets (MOPs) (Kellermann et al., 1989), which are behavioral sequences stored according to the instrumental goal to be accomplished. That is, they are schemata having to do with conventional means for accomplishing goals that are cross-situational. These sequences help us interpret the intentions of others and to translate our own goals into actions. Unlike scripts, which link situations and behaviors, scenes link goals and behaviors. Examples include action sequences for accomplishing various communicative intents, such as introducing oneself, asking permission, or engaging in conversation with a new acquaintance.

Another category of schemata has to do with *conventions of social interaction* common to multiple situations. Through years of experience in social situations and through patterns of reward and punishment in childhood and adolescence, individuals develop schemata regarding situational variables and cultural standards of communication. These internal templates tell us what is expected and appropriate within a particular social context. As outlined under the environment component, these schemata guide the selection of content and style of interaction—when and where to speak, appropriate topics in a given social situation, and appropriate nonverbal communication for the social status of the interaction partner. These overriding contextually dependent schemata have also been called managerial knowledge units (Grafman et al., 1993) and vary among cultural groups (Cole, 1989).

Table 2-4. Script for going to the doctor.

Condition for entry:	Person is sick Patient has appointment
Roles:	Physician, nurse, receptionist, patient
Relative status:	Physician superior to nurse and receptionist; nurse and physician superior to patient
Physical setting:	Physician's office with waiting room and examining room
Props:	Patient: checkbook, insurance card Physician: medical instruments, white coat Waiting room: outdated magazines
Expected behavior:	Patient: convey information to physician Physician: ask questions, examine, provide diagnosis, and prescribe treatment
Chain of events:	Patient calls to make appointment Patient goes to doctor's office before set time Patient goes to receptionist's window and signs in Patient completes forms, if initial visit Patient sits in waiting room, reads magazines Nurse comes to door of waiting room and calls patient's name Patient follows nurse to intermediate area Nurse asks what problem is Patient tells nurse presenting problem Nurse takes temperature, blood pressure, weight Nurse escorts patient to examining room Patient waits for physician in examining room Physician knocks and comes into examining room Patient tells physician presenting problem, symptoms Physician examines patient Physician tells patient the diagnosis and prescribes treatment Patient goes to receptionist area and pays for visit Patient leaves the medical office

Grice's (1975) *rules of cooperation and politeness* are a variation of this type of schemata. He states that speakers universally appear to operate with several basic principles of conversation:

A. Say only what you believe to be true or what you have evidence for.
B. Make your contribution as informative as needed, but not more informative than necessary.

C. Make your contribution relevant.

D. Be brief and orderly and avoid obscurity and ambiguity.

Conventions in the organization or semantic structure of familiar text types, called *discourse grammars*, also exist. When a person tells a narrative, the expected structure is a series of events that are temporally and causally connected, beginning with a setting, followed by a complicating action or episode, and ending with a resolution (Stein & Glenn, 1979; Ulatowska, Allard, & Chapman, 1990). Explaining how to do something, or procedural discourse, on the other hand, is organized in a temporal and hierarchical sequence of actions necessary for accomplishing a certain goal.

The role of stored knowledge in our processing and social behavior is far-reaching. Much of our comprehension, especially of nonliteral interpretations, occurs through accessing our files of stored linguistic and nonlinguistic knowledge to make appropriate implicatures and interpretations (Murphy, 1990). Stored knowledge aids in the understanding the communication of others by helping the listener fill in the gaps in information, define and organize the relationships of various elements, appreciate the feelings and experiences of others, determine the correct sense of a word when multiple meanings are possible, and anticipate what a speaker might say (Einstein, McDaniel, Bowers, & Stevens, 1984). For example, an individual who has limited schemata concerning cars and motors will have difficulty comprehending a television program or discussion on engine repair or maintenance. Without a frame of reference, processing of new information and, therefore, comprehension is limited.

Schemata also facilitate learning by providing a structure to which new information can be added. In addition they assist in developing a strategy for retrieval and in reconstructing messages by providing a basis for generating reasonable guesses (Singer, 1990).

Stored knowledge also serves as a guide for the production of social behavior. Schemata provide a framework for formulating new messages (Bracewell, Frederiksen, & Frederiksen, 1982), for planning and executing everyday activities (Bower et al., 1979), and for producing the gist of a message (Singer, 1990). The availability and use of schemata reduce the level of cognitive effort required in social situations, to the point of automatic activation in usual and customary communicative events (Kellermann et al., 1989).

Stored Knowledge Following Brain Injury

There are a number of reasons to suspect problems in the quality and adequacy of world knowledge in persons with brain injury. Many persons who sustain trauma are injured during the teenage years, a stage of development in which adult social skills begin to emerge. In addition, some individuals may have had preinjury learning or social adjustment problems that would have restricted their social and conceptual development relative to their peers, anyway.

The brain injury, itself, may have damaged the stored knowledge. Individuals who have sustained brain injury often have a reduced vocabulary (Braun, Lussier, Baribeau, & Ethier, 1989), a reduced fund of general information, and impaired word retrieval (Levin, Grossman, Sarwar, & Meyers, 1981; Sarno, 1984b). Although there is evidence that scripts for stereotypic everyday events, such as grocery shopping (Hartley & Jensen, 1991), and knowledge of narrative schemata (Liles, Coelho, Duffy, & Zalagens, 1989) may be preserved to some degree, knowledge of social conventions for politeness and for the organization of conversation may be impaired (Coelho, Liles, & Duffy, 1991a).

Several researchers have concluded that individuals with brain injury may not experience so much a loss of their world knowledge as a disruption of the organization of the knowledge base (Gruen, Frankle, & Schwartz, 1990; Levin & Goldstein, 1986; Szekeres, 1992), delayed access to stored information (Baddeley, Harris, Sunderland, Watts, & Wilson, 1987; Haut, Petros, & Frank, 1990; Tromp & Mulder, 1991), or a lack of efficient strategies for utilizing semantic memory (Hux, Beukelman, Dombrovskis, & Snyder, 1993; Levin & Goldstein, 1986). Hux et al. (1993) found that persons with TBI tended to use organizational strategies based on recent life events and personal preferences, strategies that change with time, as opposed to organizational strategies based on superordinate-subordinate relations. Although knowledge may be maintained, it is lost in a functional sense because of the lack of easy access (Tromp & Mulder, 1991). An additional factor is that accessing semantic memory appears to require greater cognitive effort for individuals with TBI (Haut, Petros, Frank, & Haut, 1991).

Cognitive Processes

The previous two components set the stage for the next component of the model. Through cognitive processes, information from the environment is continuously monitored, received, and processed by an individual during normal social interaction. In most situations, this occurs in an automatic manner. We visually scan our environment, attend to relevant features such as speech and gestures directed toward us, hold the information in memory long enough to process it, and analyze the phonological, syntactic, and semantic components of the verbal message, as well as the prosodic and spatial components of the nonverbal message.

Cognitive abilities include attention, perception, memory and learning, language, and visual-spatial perception. Hierarchical organization is characteristic of cognitive processing, in that attention is necessary for memory processing and attention and memory are basic cognitive skills that support the perception and comprehension of both linguistic and nonlinguistic input.

As discussed in the previous sections, cognitive processing is influenced by subcortical-limbic input, especially arousal, and by the knowledge base with which it can interface. The executive control center exerts control over cognitive processing, particularly in new situations or where effort is required.

Cognitive Changes Following Brain Injury

Because of the widespread, multifocal damage of closed head injury, changes in almost every aspect of cognitive functioning are found following brain injury. These changes are briefly described here. For more detailed information on normal cognitive processes and the disruptions due to brain injury the reader should check the citations listed in Table 2–5.

Attentional processes, in addition to the arousal aspects already mentioned, are affected in a number of ways by TBI. One of the most frequently reported and persisting cognitive changes after traumatic brain injury is slowed information processing, as reflected by longer reaction time and poorer performance on time-limited tasks (Ponsford & Kinsella, 1992; Tromp & Mulder, 1991; Van Zomeren, Brouwer, & Deelman, 1984). Decreased information processing capacity and speed are most evident in novel situations (Tromp & Mulder, 1991) and where decision making is required (Schmitter-Edgecombe, Marks, Fahy, & Long, 1992).

Vigilance, or the capacity to sustain a readiness to respond to a continuous and repetitive activity over a period of time (generally 30 minutes to 8 hours), has been found to be impaired in some studies (Van Zomeren, 1981) and not in others (Ponsford & Kinsella, 1992). Impaired vigilance can be the result of poor arousal or poor control over attention. Control over cognitive processes is a function of the executive control center in the model and will be discussed in the next section.

The process of memory involves the retention of input for sufficient time to process and store the information. Memory deficits are another of the more frequently reported long-term cognitive deficits following TBI, mentioned by 50% of severely injured individuals and 79% of their families as being present even 7 years postinjury (Oddy, Coughlan, Tyerman, & Jenkins, 1985). Because one must attend to information to remember it, many memory failures after TBI are actually the result of attention deficits (Wood, 1990).

Immediate recall of information is generally intact or mildly impaired by brain injury, but recall after a delay (as short as 30 minutes) is often significantly reduced (Brooks, 1975), making learning of new information

Table 2-5. References on cognitive processes and the effects of brain injury.

General Cognitive Abilities

Adamovich (1991)

Adamovich, Henderson, and Auerbach (1985)

Levin, Grafman, and Eisenberg (1987)

Lezak (1983)

Sohlberg and Mateer (1989b)

Szekeres, Ylvisaker, and Cohen (1987)

Szekeres, Ylvisaker, and Holland (1985)

Attention

Gronwall (1987)

Posner and Rafal (1987)

Van Zomeren and Brouwer (1987)

Van Zomeren, Brouwer, and Deelman (1984)

Weber (1990)

Wood (1990)

Memory

Baddeley, Harris, Sunderland, Watts, and Wilson (1987)

Wilson (1987)

Visual-Spatial Perception and Integration

Gianutsos and Matheson (1987)

Ratcliff (1987)

Language

Hagen (1984)

Hartley and Levin (1990)

Marquardt, Stoll, and Sussman (1990)

Sarno (1988)

difficult. The anterior-mesial temporal lobes and the diencephalon are areas associated with memory processes, with lateralized functions (Lezak, 1983). Left temporal lobe lesions result in a relatively specific deficit in verbal memory and learning, whereas right temporal lesions result in deficits in remembering visual information (Delany, Rosen, Mattson, & Novelly, 1980; Ojemann, 1978).

Procedural memory is the ability to learn and retain motor and pattern analyzing skills, such as riding a bicycle or mirror reading. In contrast to other types of memory, procedural learning is relatively preserved after brain injury (Ewert, Levin, Watson, & Kalisky, 1989).

Visual-spatial processing can be affected by damage to the posterior region of the right hemisphere or to the frontal lobes, which direct, organize, and regulate visual-spatial processing. Some of the problems noted after brain injury include difficulty processing facial affect (Braun, Baribeau, Ethier, Daigneault, & Proulx, 1989), poorly organized visual scanning, spatial disorientation, difficulty in perception of personal space, and difficulty interpreting complex visual information, such as pictures and maps.

The primary persisting discrete linguistic deficits after TBI are in naming, rapid word retrieval, comprehension of complex paragraphs or multistage directions, and writing to dictation (Levin et al., 1981; Sarno, 1980, 1984b). Aphasia is occasionally found and generally is associated with focal left hemisphere damage. Severe persisting general language deficits are more commonly found in conjunction with severe overall cognitive dysfunction (Levin et al., 1981). On a functional level, the most common language problems are difficulty in the comprehension and production of discourse in natural settings, in the appropriate social use of language, and in the use of language to organize and regulate cognition, learning, and behavior.

All of these changes in cognitive processes contribute to ineffective social communication following TBI. Typical cognitive changes and their effect on social communication are outlined in Table 2–6.

Executive Control Center: Prefrontal Regions

As stated before, the prefrontal regions of the brain are felt to be responsible for a number of complex functions that are at the core of our "humanness." As shown in Figure 2–1, the prefrontal regions, referred to here as the executive control center, are the point of integration of internal and external stimuli to ensure that behavior is compatible with the context and with the individual's needs. The complex nature of this adaptive function, with its multiple effects on behavior, has made it difficult to formulate one model of frontal lobe functioning. Several models have been hypothesized (Goldman-Rakic, 1993; Grafman et al., 1993; Lezak, 1993; Luria, 1973; Shallice & Burgess, 1991; Stuss, 1991). Reviews of literature regarding the various aspects of frontal lobe functioning can be found in Daigneault, Braun, and Whitaker (1992); Hart and Jacobs (1993); Levin, Eisenberg, and Benton (1991); and Mattson and Levin (1990). Ylvisaker (1992) reviews the contributions of frontal lobe dysfunction to cognitive-communicative abilities following TBI. Table 2–7 lists the various functions that have been attributed to the prefrontal lobe regions from the above sources.

One of the major roles of the frontal lobes is to regulate cognitive processes. In this role, normal frontal lobe functioning ensures the efficient allocation of attentional resources in a goal-directed fashion, particularly in new or complex situations. The frontal system can activate the lower arousal system when increased mental effort or divided attention is re-

Table 2–6.   Linguistic, cognitive, and executive/behavioral changes after brain injury and their effects on social communication.

Area	Changes Due to Brain Injury	Effects on Social Communication
Language	Reduced comprehension as length, complexity, or rate increases Reduced vocabulary, especially for multiple meanings and context of usage Decreased naming Reduced word fluency Reduced comprehension of abstract language	Difficulty comprehending normal rate of conversation Difficulty following directions Problem with use of word in appropriate semantic context Problems understanding abstract meanings of words, idiomatic expressions, or proverbs Hesitations or filled pauses in discourse due to delayed word retrieval Selection of inappropriate word or vague term; circumlocution Difficulty getting to the point
Attention/Concentration Arousal/Alertness	Decreased orienting response Lapses in alertness	Difficulty orienting to stimulus and attending at beginning of interaction Difficulty staying on topic and maintaining interaction Appearance of disinterest in others Limited eye gaze and verbal feedback to speaker Slurred speech
Sustained Attention/Vigilance	Inconsistent attention to ongoing stimulus Lapses in attention	Inconsistent perception of words or spatial information Topic change without warning
Selective Attention	Difficulty filtering out irrelevant stimuli Distractibility Poor concentration Poor attention to more than one task or stimulus at a time	Difficulty comprehending and speaking in situations with distractions, noises or when more than one partner involved Difficulty maintaining consistent point of view, intent, topic Rambling or tangential discourse Difficulty talking or listening if doing another task

Continued

Table 2–6.   *Continued*

Area	Changes Due to Brain Injury	Effects on Social Communication
Flexibility/Shifting Attention	Difficulty shifting attention as needed	Difficulty switching topics, listener/speaker role Difficulty comprehending context when a sudden change occurs
Speed of Processing	Slowed information processing Slowness in encoding social situation Slowness in decision making	Long pauses within discourse or before responding Slowed rate of speaking Difficulty comprehending normal rate of speech Difficulty staying on topic in a group discussion
Visuospatial Perception	Misperception of complex visual information Disorganized scanning of environment Misperception of environmental cues or nonverbal communication Spatial disorientation	Difficulty with spatial terms in directions or conversation Difficulty detecting feelings, intent of others Inappropriate choice of style, time, or place for a given context Invasion of personal space of partner
Memory/Learning	Poor short-term memory Susceptibility to interference in learning Intrusions, embellishment, confabulation Failure to organize input for storage Failure to actively search memory Failure to apply strategies	Repetition of ideas, statements, whole conversations or stories Loss of purpose or topic of conversation Impaired recall of shared knowledge Instructions or messages forgotten or mixed up Problem staying on topic, being concise Difficulty acquiring or improving social skills through routine interactions Disorganized discourse Difficulty integrating information heard Addition of false information in conversation Limited information provided when questioned

Executive Control Center

Organization	Decreased use of organizational strategies	Decreased ability to detect main ideas, organization of information
		Poorly organized discourse or behavior
		Difficulty sequencing verbal directions
Social Inference/ Abstract Attitude	Increased focus on self	Interruption of conversations of others
	Decreased empathy	Use of rude or inappropriate remarks
	Difficulty inferring social and cognitive context	Excessive talking about personal experiences or feelings
	Decreased perspective taking	Inability to adapt style and information to partner's need/ context
		Inflexibility in opinions, attitudes
		Difficulty understanding feelings, motivations, opinions of others
		Immature communication style
		Difficulty expressing concern for others
		Difficulty detecting intent of speaker
		Use of nonspecific reference
		Poor generalization of skills
Synthesis/Integration	Difficulty integrating verbal and nonverbal information	Difficulty using a map, giving or taking directions
	Difficulty synthesizing multiple sources of information	Difficulty detecting contradictory verbal and nonverbal communication
	Difficulty integrating input with prior knowledge	Difficulty incorporating contextual cues into communication
		Difficulty making inferences, seeing relationships between ideas
		Fragmented explanations or descriptions
		Mismatch between verbal and nonverbal message

Continued

Table 2-6. Continued

Area	Changes Due to Brain Injury	Effects on Social Communication
Initiation/Formulation of Goal	Reduced drive Reduced initiation Reduced motivation	Flattened affect Reduced range of emotional features of communication, both in body language and paralinguistic features Difficulty making effort to attend or participate when needed Lack of spontaneity in interactions Appearance of disinterest in others Difficulty initiating and maintaining conversation Limited use of questions or expanded remarks in conversations Failure to seek information from others, to pursue friendships Failure to seek clarification when comprehension breaks down
Planning/Sequencing	Poor motor sequencing Decreased planning	Lack of coherence, organization to discourse Fractured approach to interactions Inclusion of excessive detail in discourse Excessive revisions, false starts in discourse
Carrying Out Plans	Poor follow-through Perseveration Impersistence	Lack of consistency between what person says and what actually does Tangential discourse Stereotypic responses Difficulty maintaining one purpose in interaction Inability to use language to direct behavior
Monitoring and Self-Correction	Poor error recognition Poor use of feedback Poor monitoring of behavior	Failure to monitor own comprehension and ask for clarification Lack of response to nonverbal cues of partner regarding level of interest or understanding

Regulation of Behavior and Emotions	Disinhibition Excessive display of emotion	Difficulty adjusting speech rate, loudness, intelligibility to fit context Failure to self-correct inconsistencies or errors Inappropriate laughter Excessive talking Use of inappropriate sexual comments Excessive friendliness, talking with strangers Excessive complaining, expression of anger Nonpurposeful behavior or speech that is distracting to self and others Initiation of unnecessary questions Unpredictable social behavior
Problem Solving/ Anticipation	Poor anticipation of consequences Poor ability to recognize when problem exists Decreased ability to brainstorm solutions, evaluate possibilities, implement solution and evaluate process	Frustration in interpersonal situations or withdrawal when conflict occurs Difficulty resolving conflicts Use of aggressive or passive responses Lack of foresight Immature style in conflicts
Self-Awareness/ Metacognition	Difficulty assessing personal strengths and needs Unrealistic goal setting	Lack of credibility with others Attempts unrealistic life situations or goals Failure to employ compensatory strategies to improve communication

Continued

Table 2–6. *Continued*

Area	Changes Due to Brain Injury	Effects on Social Communication
Abstract Reasoning	Failure to generate or use strategies to improve	Resistance to "help" from others
		Failures attributed to others
	Decreased abstract reasoning	Failure to take into account facts not immediately present
	Poor judgment	Decreased comprehension of abstract language, humor, indirect requests
		Difficulty making inferences, drawing conclusions from discourse
		Inappropriate requests of others
		Difficulty evaluating validity of information, reasoning of others
		Concrete interpretation of vocabulary or message
		Difficulty applying new learning

Table 2-7.   Functions associated with the prefrontal lobe regions.

Control of attentional processes

Control of memory

Regulation of drives and impulses

Regulation of emotions

Working memory

Integration of input and output

Social perception

Empathy/Abstract attitude

Goal formulation

Planning and sequencing behavior

Initiation of goal-directed behavior

Monitoring and evaluating

Abstract thinking

Judgment

Problem solving

Anticipation of future events/estimation

Self-awareness

Verbal mediation of behavior

Metacognition

quired. It helps maintain attention and concentration, inhibiting attention to irrelevant or redundant sensory information. It controls the focusing and shifting of attention. The frontal lobes influence attention through extensive bidirectional connections with the reticular activating system and the diencephalon and connections with the primary sensory areas of the brain.

Control of memory processes by the prefrontal regions is demonstrated in several ways. The frontal system organizes input for more efficient learning, suppresses interference, generates strategies to enhance the storage and retrieval of information, and integrates new material with old knowledge.

The frontal lobes influence visual-spatial processing by ensuring the drive and attention needed for processing relevant features, by organizing the input, and by synthesizing the visual information and integrating it with past knowledge and with verbal input. The influence of the frontal lobes on language and cognition and the resulting effects in functional communication are outlined in Table 2–6.

The frontal lobes also modulate and regulate the expression of internal drives and affective states, so that satisfaction of needs considers the social environment and social and cultural constraints on behavior. The mesial temporal lobe, hypothalamus, and other limbic structures have projections to and from the frontal cortex, particularly the ventromedial region (Eslinger & Damasio, 1985).

The prefrontal region also has been posited as the source of "working memory," a mechanism for integrating sensory information with internal knowledge to guide interpretation of ongoing interactions, to organize information, to determine the appropriate synthesis of information, and to plan a response (Goldman-Rakic, 1993; Hart & Jacobs, 1993). By doing so, the prefrontal region provides continuity and coherence to our thinking and communication.

Certain roles of the frontal lobe have been called the "executive functions" (Lezak, 1982; 1987a; 1993). These include goal setting, behavior planning and sequencing, goal-oriented behavior initiation, self-monitoring, and evaluation of behavior. These roles can be incorporated into the "working memory" concept, in that information regarding the environment and the internal drives, motivation, and mood must be integrated to form a plan of action related to a goal and then the plan must be monitored in working memory and adapted as needed.

A part of this executive control is the initiation of an active search for an appropriate script or apposition for a given situation from semantic memory. A determination must be made regarding the fit between the schema and the available input regarding the communicative context. Conscious monitoring of the selected schema by the control center once it is put into play is necessary to assess ongoing effectiveness and appropriateness as an interaction evolves. This ability relies on adequate social perception and inferences, but may be conducted in a fairly automatic manner in routine, everyday situations.

Problem solving and abstract thinking are also functions associated with the frontal lobes. Problem solving requires the ability to adequately perceive the social and physical environment, anticipate consequences of possible responses, control impulses and emotional responses for selection of the most appropriate solution, and make social inferences regarding the perspectives of others. It also requires the executive skills of planning, executing, monitoring, and evaluating the solution that is selected.

Abstract thinking involves going beyond a concrete interpretation to synthesize information and to apply stored knowledge. This is necessary to determine the gist of a message, to infer relationships, and to appreciate abstract linguistic forms, such as indirect requests, humor, idiomatic expressions, and proverbs.

Social inferential ability is the ability to perceive and interpret the feelings and thoughts of others (McTear & Conti-Ramsden, 1992). Socially adept individuals must be able to recognize the emotional and cognitive status of a listener and adjust their messages to the listener. This ability appears to a prefrontal function.

The ability to see oneself clearly, or "self-awareness," and metacognition are additional functions of the frontal lobe. Self-awareness involves realistic appraisal of one's own strengths and needs. Metacognition refers to the capacity to reflect on one's own cognitive abilities, to understand that there are ways of improving those abilities, and to purposefully employ strategies to enhance one's abilities. Luria (1973) hypothesizes that the frontal lobes are responsible for the verbal mediation of behavior and cognition and asserts that the frontal lobes are the source of our "self talk" or "inner speech."

Executive Functioning Following Brain Injury

Problems in the executive control center are common following closed head injury not only because of the high frequency of frontal lobe damage, but also from the characteristic diffuse axonal damage. This white matter damage may cause a functional disconnection of frontal lobe control from its subcortical and cortical projections.

It has been hypothesized that there are two major patterns of disruption in the regulation of cognition and affective and social behavior after TBI (Auerbach, 1986). As summarized in Table 2–8, individuals with orbitofrontal damage tend to demonstrate "excess" in all areas. They are impulsive and unable to inhibit internal drives and thoughts (disinhibition) or external stimulation (distractibility). They exhibit poor control over emotional input and may be irritable, even violent, unrealistically happy, or labile. They tend to talk excessively with tangential content and demonstrate poor social perception and difficulty following social rules.

In contrast, individuals who have sustained dorsolateral damage demonstrate an "impoverished" picture of cognition and behavior. These individuals lack the ability to formulate and initiate goal-directed behavior. Drive may be diminished to the point that expression of any emotion or desire is lacking. Thinking and comprehension are concrete, with limited language output or social interaction. Motor sequencing difficulty and decreased mental flexibility are common. Problems in maintaining and shifting mental sets are characteristic as well.

Lateralized effects of frontal injuries also have been found (see review in Mattson & Levin, 1990). As listed in Table 2–9, left frontal damage results in increased personal concern and depression, with decreased initiation, particularly in verbal output. Right frontal damage has been associated with unawareness, inability to read social cues including prosody, difficulty producing appropriate nonverbal modes of communication, prob-

Table 2–8.   Characteristic behaviors associated with orbitofrontal and dorsolateral frontal damage.

Orbitofrontal	Dorsolateral
Poor social judgment	Reduced initiation
Impulsivity	Apathy
Disinhibition	Lack of drive
Lack of concern for others	Lack of emotion
Euphoria	Decreased anticipation
Sexual disinhibition	Impoverished discourse
Restlessness	Concrete thinking
Lability	Perseveration
Talkativeness	Decreased working memory
"Pseudopsychopathic" personality	"Pseudodepressed" personality
Irritability	Slowness
Distractibility	Difficulty forming and shifting mental sets
Loss of control of anger	Decreased mental flexibility
	Motor sequencing difficulty

Table 2–9.   Lateralized deficits associated with prefrontal lobe damage.

Left Prefrontal Damage	Right Prefrontal Damage
Increased personal concern	Unawareness
Depression	Inability to read social cues
Decreased initiation	Inability to produce appropriate nonverbal communication
Decreased verbal fluency	
Reduced language output	Decreased comprehension of prosody and indirect intents/meanings
	Inattention to context
	Increased anxiety

lems interpreting indirect intents and meanings, increased anxiety, and inattention to context.

Some of the major effects of frontal lobe dysfunction on social communication are listed in Table 2–6. As discussed under the section on environment, persons with brain injuries frequently appear to demonstrate difficulty using contextual information in their comprehension and production of communication. In addition to the possible explanations previously mentioned, this difficulty in social perception might be caused by a reduced capacity of working memory—difficulty holding multiple forms of input for integration necessary for the synthesis of nonverbal and verbal aspects of a message or integration of stored knowledge with cognitive and perceptual data. Researchers with other populations have speculated that inadequate "on-line" integration of knowledge during listening contributes to poor comprehension of what others say (Royer & Cunningham, 1981), to poor understanding of figurative language, and to failure to draw accurate inferences (Dennis & Lovett, 1990).

Another causal factor may be a speaker's inability to appreciate the significance of contextual cues or to take the listener's perspective. In other words, due to problems in executive functions such as integration of multiple types of information, monitoring, or assumption of an abstract attitude, an individual makes inappropriate assumptions about a social situation or a listener's knowledge base or shared knowledge or focus of attention. He or she may not be able to get beyond a concrete interpretation of a situation or to make social inferences. For example, a therapist, noticing that an individual still had on her heavy jacket in the middle of a therapy session, asked "Jane, do you want your jacket on?" to indirectly ask if she wanted to take off the jacket. The client's response was a puzzled look at the therapist with the statement, "I already have it on."

Comprehension of Social Communication

The comprehension of functional communication requires that each previously mentioned component of the model in Figure 2–1 participate in making sense of the verbal and nonverbal input from the environment. The contribution of each component of the model to comprehension has already been elaborated, and this section summarizes the nature of comprehension failure after brain injury. (Also see Table 2–6.)

To establish the correct "listener" set, an individual must be motivated and receptive to interaction with other persons. After brain injury, the drive to make an effort may be diminished or the mood or emotional state may preclude active listening, especially when greater effort is needed or when the individual has no personal interest in a topic.

Arousal and attentional problems may interfere with reception of adequate input, especially in the midst of noisy or distracting environments typical of everyday situations. Conversations require the shifting of attention as speakers and topics change. Reduced speed of processing may mean that an individual is not able to keep up with a typical rate of conversation. Attention may be directed to insignificant details or stimuli unrelated to a conversation, resulting in skewed comprehension of discourse or social interaction. An individual's slow processing may make it difficult to shift between speaking and listening roles.

Memory problems also prevent adequate understanding. An individual may not retain what was said at the beginning of a conversation or remember the topic. In some situations, individuals forget their current location and why they are there, inserting confusion into the situation. Temporal marking of memories may also be impaired, making it difficult to establish a memory for a sequence of events or who said what in which order. It is difficult to make sense of a conversation or an event when there is no continuity of memory.

When visuospatial processing or executive problems are present, situational cues for discourse meaning may not be detected by an individual with TBI or cues may not be used to make sense of the verbal message. Difficulty with comprehension of prosody may be experienced as well.

Changes in the executive control center can have a number of additional effects on comprehension. Without effective organizational strategies or sufficient working memory capacity, an individual is not able to adequately comprehend discourse because of failure to detect main ideas or separate details from main ideas. Input is often not integrated into the existing knowledge base, so the individual is not able to see the relevance of information, infer relationships, or retain the information. Due to problems in abstract reasoning, interpretation of abstract or figurative language and inferential reasoning are poor. Changes in social inferential ability may lead to misjudgments about the intent of others, inability to detect deception, sarcasm, false promises, or jokes (McTear & Conti-Ramsden, 1992).

Communication Behaviors

As stated before, communication behaviors are a set of social behaviors (Prutting, 1982). There is no one way to catalog or study social behavior. Some approaches employ molar analyses of behavior, such as overall ratings of social skill, social anxiety, or social competence (Newton & Johnson, 1985), with others measuring molecular level responses, such as length of eye gaze or time spent smiling. Prutting and Kirchner (1983, 1987), Roth and Spekman (1984), and McTear (1985) offer taxonomies at a more intermediate level of analysis. As shown in Table 2–10, three major types of social communicative behaviors are generally included: nonverbal, interactional, and propositional aspects of communication. Although behaviors associated with greater social skill are highlighted here, it should be remembered that acceptable communication behaviors are defined by an individual's cultural background (Cole, 1989). Therefore, judgments regarding appropriateness of social behavior must consider the cultural environment of an individual.

Table 2-10. Categories of communicative behaviors.

Nonverbal aspects of communication
  Paralinguistic features
  Kinesics
  Proxemics

Interactional aspects of communication
  Turn taking
  Conversational repair
  Speech acts

Propositional aspects of communication
  Topic management
  Informativeness
  Cohesion
  Semantic plan

Nonverbal Aspects of Communication

Some experts have estimated that up to 93% of what we communicate in interpersonal interactions is through nonverbal means, through paralinguistics, kinesics, or proxemics (Mehrabian, 1968).

Paralinguistic features of communication are inherent aspects of speech production, such as vocal quality, loudness, speech intelligibility, fluency or ease of production, and prosody. Prosody is the combination of patterns of changes in pitch, loudness, and rate that result in intonation contours and syllabic and word stress. Paralinguistic features convey information about the personality, emotional state, and physical features of the speaker. They also function to augment the propositional content by indicating the type of utterance (e.g., inflection indicating a statement versus a question) or by stressing key or new information in the message. In sarcasm, paralinguistic features are used to indicate that the intended meaning is the opposite of the propositional content (e.g., "Well, he was a big help!").

Kinesics is communication through body movements, including facial expressions, eye gaze, general body posture, and gestures. These behaviors are used to substitute for a verbal response, to augment or complement a verbal response, or to assist in the regulation of conversational turns. Eye gaze and facial expression are used by listeners to indicate the level of understanding and to encourage or discourage social interaction. Generally, individuals who use more smiling, greater eye contact, a mobile and open body posture, and frequent, appropriate gestures are perceived as having greater social competence (Liberman, 1982).

Proxemics is defined as the use and perception of social and personal space in communication. The context of the communication, the relationship of the partners, and cultural norms determine the acceptable interpersonal distance and use of touching or physical contact. Individuals who have their personal space invaded without permission generally feel violated and uncomfortable in the social interaction.

Nonverbal Communication Following Brain Injury

Although descriptions of communication and other social behaviors after brain injury suggest that many problems exist in nonverbal communication, only a few studies have evaluated this area. Milton et al. (1984) used the Pragmatic Protocol of Prutting and Kirchner (1983) to examine the videotaped conversational interactions of five individuals with brain injury. Prosody was the pragmatic behavior most frequently judged to be inappropriate, with all five persons demonstrating problems in this area. Problems in affect control, such as excessive laughter, were noted in four of the five subjects. Inappropriate fluency and intelligibility were demonstrated by two of the five subjects despite the absence of dysarthria.

Hartley and Jensen (1991) found that, as a group, individuals with brain injury demonstrated greater problems in fluency; they spoke at a slower rate of speech and with more dysfluencies than did noninjured speakers. Patterns of variation, however, were noted. Some individuals with brain injury spoke at a much slower rate of speech and used long, unfilled pauses but few dysfluencies, with others speaking at a close to normal rate but demonstrating many dysfluencies (Hartley & Jensen, 1992).

Marsh and Knight (1991) had two observers (psychologists) rate the social communication of 18 individuals with severe brain injury and 18 control subjects on six 7-point rating scales. The subjects with brain injuries were consistently rated as being more inappropriate on the speech delivery scale that incorporated paralinguistic features (speech fluency, rate of speech, and voice quality), as compared with the control subjects.

In a study of coverbal or kinesic behaviors, Katz, LaPointe, and Markel (1978) found only minimal differences between persons with aphasia and normal speakers. The individuals with aphasia, however, did tend to engage in several behaviors, such as head shakes and head nods, for a longer period of time—generally to indicate a desire to continue speaking.

Interactional Aspects of Communication

The second major category of social communication behaviors covers interactional aspects of communication. These behaviors reflect the reciprocal nature of conversation and the joint cooperation required of the participants (McTear, 1985). *Turn taking* is the most obvious example; conversations are organized so that participants initiate and give turns with a minimum of overlaps or gaps (Sacks, Schegloff, & Jefferson, 1974). Turn taking is a skilled activity that is based on an intricate set of rules requiring linguistic and pragmatic knowledge. Conversational turns are locally governed, with each turn contingent on the preceding utterance or situation. The length, content, and order of turns are not specified in advance. Turn taking is signaled through eye gaze, prosody, and pauses. Skilled participants shift easily from speaker to listener roles without remaining too long in either mode (McTear & Conti-Ramsden, 1992). Precisely timed turn taking requires rapid processing and production of language (McTear & Conti-Ramsden, 1992).

Conversational repair is the second behavior that reflects the interactional nature of social interaction; in both listener and speaker roles, participants have a responsibility to initiate repair when communication breakdown occurs. A speaker is expected not only to attempt to produce an accurate message, but also to perceive when the listener might not understand and to initiate repair through repetition, clarification, or revision. For example, a speaker might respond to a listener's puzzled look by providing more specific directions or restating the request in a louder tone of voice. It is the listener's responsibility to indicate his or her level of understanding and to request repair if needed, either by posing questions or by asking for repetition or clarification.

A third way of viewing conversational interactions is by analyzing the *communicative intent* or the purpose of each turn. This process highlights that we communicate with a goal in mind, whether it be to direct someone's behavior, to make a comment, to ask for information (Searle, 1969), or just to maintain interpersonal relationships (Liberman, 1982). Taxonomies of communicative intents (also called speech acts), such as the one in Table 2–11, generally include the categories of ritualizing, requesting and giving information, controlling, and expressing and responding to attitudes or feelings (Searle, 1969; Wiig, 1982a, 1982b). The term *social skills* from the psychological literature often has the same meaning as speech acts (see Goldstein, Sprafkin, Gershaw, & Klein, 1980), but generally encompasses a broader range of behaviors, including nonverbal aspects of communication.

Competent communicators are able to use language to accomplish a variety of intents. The ability to use a variety of speech acts, to understand the intent of an utterance, and to respond with an act that matches the speech act of the preceding utterance (e.g., a question is followed by an answer) is generally acquired by adolescence (Allen & Brown, 1976).

Interactional Aspects Following Brain Injury

Individuals who have sustained a brain injury frequently demonstrate problems with the interactional nature of conversation. In their study, Milton et al. (1984) found that three of the five (60%) adults with brain injury had

Table 2-11.   A taxonomy of speech acts or social skills.

Ritualizing
Greets others
Introduces self
Starts a conversation

Asking for/giving information
Requests/tells name, phone number, address
Requests/gives description

Controlling behavior of others
Asks for favors or assistance
Makes a complaint/criticism
Gives instructions or directions
Tries to persuade/convince others

Expressing feelings
Gives/accepts an apology
Expresses agreement or disagreement

Imagining

problems initiating turns, taking turns without excessive pause time, and relating each turn to the preceding utterance. A restricted repertoire of speech acts, or social skills, immature or socially inappropriate use of speech acts, and difficulty detecting the intent of the speaker are problems that have been described by clinicians (Braunling-McMorrow, Lloyd, & Fralish, 1986; Ehrlich & Sipes, 1985).

Marsh and Knight (1991) report that their subjects who had sustained a brain injury were rated more deficient than noninjured speakers on a social interaction scale measuring partner-directed behavior. That is, persons with brain injuries frequently failed to initiate as much interaction, to use reinforcers during their partner's conversational turn, and to show interest in their partner. Similar results were obtained by Coelho et al. (1991a). The individuals with TBI in this study had problems initiating turns in conversation, tending to respond to requests or questions of the communication partner with adequate but minimal responses without making efforts to facilitate the continuation of conversation.

Propositional Aspects of Communication

The third major category of social communication, or pragmatic, behaviors examines the propositional content of the communication and includes the notions of relevancy, clarity of reference, and coherence. This category has to do with the manner in which discourse is organized with respect to an overall plan, theme, or topic and how individual utterances are conceptually linked to maintain unity. More specifically, topic management, informativeness, cohesion, and discourse organization are included in this category.

Topic management is a key component of well-formed, or coherent, discourse (Mentis & Prutting, 1991; Scinto, 1977; van Dijk, 1977). A competent speaker is able to select topics that are appropriate and relevant to the conversational context and to introduce new topics in an appropriate manner. The ongoing nature of conversation requires that participants give more than minimal responses and maintain the topic by producing responses that expand or contribute to the topic. Any changes in topic must be marked in some manner, such as saying, "Oh, by the way, ..." A competent communicator does not dominate a conversation through the number of topics initiated, but rather cooperates for an equal balance (Wiemann, 1977).

The term *informativeness* denotes variations in the amount and form of content based on assumptions about shared knowledge and the needs of a listener. A speaker must be able to appreciate the perspective of a communication partner to determine the quantity of information and specificity of referents in a particular situation to convey thoughts without ambiguity or redundancy. Sufficient information must be given for effective communication, with the most important information highlighted and new information distinguished from old.

Linguistic devices such as deixis and cohesion, including direct/indirect reference, are examples of instances in which role-taking ability is necessary. *Deictic terms* are words whose interpretations are based on the external context of the communication, such as, the physical setting, the participants, and the relative time. For example, the referents for the pronouns *I* and *you* change depending on the person speaking at a given time. Demonstrative pronouns (*this, that*), when used in utterances such as "Please pick that up," are understood, based on the shared physical setting and the nonverbal cues of the speaker. The meaning of certain adverbs of location (e.g., *here, there*) and prepositions (e.g., *in front of, behind*) is determined by the location of the speaker and/or listener (e.g., Here is your lunch; Put this behind the tree). Certain verbs, such as *come, go, bring,* and *take,* are also deictic terms, because selection depends on the location of the participants.

Cohesive ties are words in the surface structure of a discourse that tie the meanings of sentences together (Halliday & Hasan, 1976). They involve presupposition, in that interpretation of one linguistic element relies on another element in the discourse. Halliday and Hasan (1976) outline five major categories of cohesion: reference, substitution, ellipsis, conjunction, and lexical. Reference cohesive ties include personal and demonstrative pronouns and indirect/direct reference (*a* versus *the*) and are the most frequently occurring type of cohesion in narratives (Hartley & Jensen, 1991; Mentis & Prutting, 1987). The following two utterances illustrate several types of cohesive ties:

Bob lost his keys/*or* at least *he* thought he *did/*

Or is a conjunction and is used not only to tie the two utterances together, but also to indicate that the second will somehow contradict the first. *He* is a personal pronoun that cannot be interpreted unless one makes reference to the previous sentence to recover the man's name, *Bob*. *Did* is an example of substitution in that *did* is a substitute for the verb phrase *lost his keys*.

In addition to having a central topic or theme and intersentential devices (cohesion) for providing connectivity, a discourse must also be organized, following an *overall goal or plan*. When telling a story, the speaker is expected to follow the narrative grammar—to provide a setting first before developing the episodes. Narrative ability also requires going beyond the literal meaning of sentences. It requires the ability to use knowledge of contexts of communication, use abstract reasoning, infer feelings and motivations, and synthesize and organize multiple pieces of information into a coherent whole.

The ability to use *abstract language* forms is another aspect of propositional behavior. These behaviors require interpretive skills that interconnect language and cognitive skills. These include the appreciation and use of humor and jokes, plus comprehension and use of figurative language, such as metaphors, idiomatic expressions, and proverbs.

Propositional Aspects Following Brain Injury

Research on discourse production after brain injury indicates that problems in topic management and degree of informativeness are common. Milton et al. (1984) note that three of their five individuals with TBI demonstrated inappropriate pragmatic behavior in the areas of topic selection, topic maintenance, and quantity/conciseness of their conversation. Mentis and Prutting (1991) conducted an extensive analysis of topic with one subject with brain injury and one control subject. The person with brain injury produced noncoherent topic changes; ambiguous, unrelated, and incomplete ideational units; fewer new information ideational units; and more passes and agreement/acknowledgment units than did the normal speaker. Similarly, Coehlo et al. (1991a) find that individuals with brain injury provide shorter, less elaborated contributions to a topic, more often leaving it to the communication partner to introduce, develop, and extend a topic of conversation.

Hartley and Jensen (1991) find that, as a group, persons with brain injuries provide fewer key content units and more inaccurate or vague information in narrative and procedural discourse than typical speakers.

Variation in performance, however, was characteristic of the group with brain injury. Some individuals provided too much detail and spoke longer than required, with other individuals providing only short utterances and drastically reduced information (Hartley & Jensen, 1992).

In addition to problems in the quantity of information content, problems in specificity of reference are also present after brain injury. Greater use of pronouns without referents as well as vague terminology or phrases are found (Hartley & Jensen, 1991; Liles et al., 1989; Mentis & Prutting, 1987).

Individuals with brain injury have been found by several investigators to use significantly fewer cohesive ties per utterance than normal speakers in narrative and procedural discourse (Hartley & Jensen, 1991; Mentis & Prutting, 1987) but not in conversational discourse (Mentis & Prutting, 1987). Other researchers found no difference between the two groups of speakers (Glosser & Deser, 1990; Liles et al., 1989).

Several investigators have hypothesized that acquired brain injury would cause problems at the macrostructure level of discourse or with discourse organization or structure, because of the cognitive and executive skills required at this level of production. Nine subjects with a fluent language disorder after acquired brain injury examined by Glosser and Deser (1990) were rated to be significantly lower in their global coherence as compared to noninjured individuals or individuals with fluent aphasia. Three of the four subjects with brain injury of Liles et al. (1989) used fewer episodes in generating a story than control speakers.

Grooming and appearance are not typically thought of as aspects of communicative behavior but have a tremendous impact on the way a person is evaluated by others in social situations (Ylvisaker, Urbanczyk, & Feeney, 1992). Poor grooming may cause the individual to be interpreted as mentally incompetent, socially withdrawn, or apathetic. This can lead to rejection in work, school, and leisure activities. Frontal lobe dysfunction often leads to decreased initiation and monitoring of effective grooming skills. Because of the impact on communicative effectiveness, grooming and appearance need to be considered in a rehabilitation setting.

Additional Considerations

Influences on social communication that are not represented in Figure 2–1 deserve attention. One major consideration is sensation; changes in sensation impact cognitive abilities and should not be completely ignored in the explanation of social communication abilities. For example, changes in visual acuity and hearing would have significant consequences on a person's ability to perceive environmental cues in social situations, understand what others say, and develop an experientially derived knowledge base.

A second factor that should be considered but is not included in the model is endurance. Fatigue is frequently reported by individuals after brain injury, even those without obvious motor system involvement. Like all of us, individuals with a brain injury can become fatigued and experience difficulty in processing information, in overall arousal/motivation, and in emotional status or coping ability. The extra effort required in social and cognitive activities after a brain injury can lead to mental, if not physical, fatigue.

A third factor not specified in the model presented in this chapter is motor skill. Obvious physical impairments often affect our perceptions of the capabilities of an individual, whereas the lack of apparent physical abnormalities makes it difficult for individuals with frontal lobe dysfunction to be perceived as having a significant disability. In addition, limitations in speech production and gestural or body control hamper the execution of skilled social behavior.

These three factors—sensation, endurance, and motor abilities—need to be considered in the evaluation and treatment of cognitive-communication disorders after brain injury. Nevertheless, the elements will not be addressed in this book, which focuses on cognitive and linguistic processing issues.

Summary

This chapter presented a model of social communication, based on a review of literature from multiple fields of study. Communication, one aspect of human social behavior, involves the interaction of a person with his or her environment. Factors within the person that influence communication include stored knowledge, cognitive processing ability, arousal, motivation, emotional status, and frontal lobe functioning. This last category includes the multiple functions of a higher level control and integration center. Functions include control of our cognitive processes, integration of multiple input, initiation of goal-directed behavior, organization of input and output processes, and evaluation and modulation of one's own behavior.

The model provides a theoretical basis for the analysis of communicative competence following brain injury. Because any or all of these areas can be affected by brain injury, evaluation strategies must consider all components of social or communication competency. The interaction and combined effect of the components are more crucial to understanding social communication than any single element. A comprehensive, integrated, and theoretically based approach to evaluation of cognitive-communicative abilities, based on this model, can now be developed.

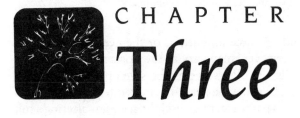

CHAPTER

Three

Functional Approaches to Assessment of Cognitive-Communicative Abilities

Natural language usage, as described in Chapter 2, is a complex, dynamic process that is characterized by both individual and situational variation among all individuals, but particularly after brain injury. The multiple variables affecting the expression of changes following traumatic brain injury (TBI) were described in Chapters 1 and 2. It should be apparent, therefore, that the evaluation of functional communication following brain injury must be a complex, multifaceted effort that is adapted to each individual to capture his or her strengths and needs, plus environmental influences on performance. Input must be obtained from multiple sources and across a variety of situations and settings to generate an ecologically valid profile of an individual. In a functional approach, an evaluation focuses on an individual's perspectives, values, goals, and needs to plan socially relevant rehabilitation for that person.

To form a holistic picture of an individual's capabilities and current functioning, input from multiple disciplines is preferred. Because of the possibility of funding and resource limitations or the needs of the client, the rehabilitation team, however, may vary at the postacute stage. Some speech-language pathologists (SLPs) serve as the sole providers of treatment at that point; other SLPs may be part of a limited team, with others fortunate enough to work as part of an interdisciplinary team offering a full complement of viewpoints and expertise. In an interdisciplinary team approach, there is close communication regarding assessment findings and treatment planning. Evaluation procedures are shared and treatment goals are collaboratively developed and implemented. On the other hand, if the involvement of other service providers is limited, the role of the speech-language pathologist in assessment and treatment will be expanded.

In any case, it should be clear that no *one* format, protocol, or battery of cognitive and communication tests can be used to evaluate individuals who have sustained brain injury. Each clinician must consider his or her setting and the person served. The evaluation process, nevertheless, should proceed in an orderly and well-conceived manner, driven by a broad view of communication with a sound theoretical foundation.

Overview of the Evaluation Process

Purposes of an Evaluation

An evaluation should be conducted to serve a number of purposes. These include to evaluate the current cognitive-communicative functioning, to develop a profile of the strengths and needs of an individual, to determine the ability to benefit from intervention, to acquire information necessary for treatment planning, and to educate an individual and significant others about the findings.

To develop a comprehensive profile of an individual's current level of functioning, the evaluator should investigate each of the variables that contribute to individual differences after brain injury. These factors were first articulated in Chapter 1 and are listed in Figure 3–1. They include the individual's preinjury level of functioning, the effects of the neurological damage on the individual's cognitive-communicative functioning, the individual's adjustment to the injury, and the influence of the social, cultural, and physical environment, plus the medical and rehabilitation history to that point.

Levels of Outcome Evaluation

Figure 3–1 also indicates that outcomes after brain injury influenced by the above factors can be assessed at several levels. The World Health Organ-

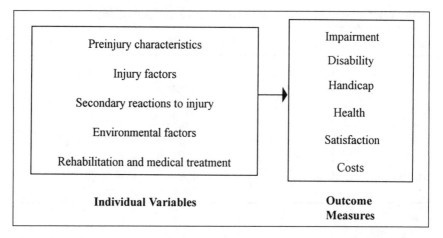

Figure 3-1. Individual variables that contribute to outcome after brain injury. (Note: From "Outcome Evaluation and Spinal Cord Injury" by G. G. Whiteneck, 1992, *Neuro Rehabilitation*, 2(4), p. 43. Copyright 1992 by Butterworth-Heinemann. Adapted by permission.)

ization's (WHO) (1980) classification of the effects of disease or injury on a person lists three levels: impairment, disability, and handicap. A differing set of terminology was proposed by Nagi (1969) and is currently favored. The WHO levels have been relabeled impairment, functional limitation, and disability.

An *impairment* exists when there is a loss or abnormality of cognitive, emotional, physiological, or anatomical structure or function. As shown in Table 3-1, examples of cognitive-communicative impairment after brain include decreased memory, reduced auditory comprehension, word-finding deficits, and reduced speed of processing. Standardized neuropsychological and language batteries typically assess at the impairment level.

Disability in the WHO classification or *functional limitation* in Nagi's model is "any restriction or lack (resulting from an impairment) of ability to perform an activity in the manner or within the range considered normal for a human being" (WHO, 1980, p. 143). Disabilities are determined by assessing the effect of impairments on functional life activities, such as mobility, psychosocial functioning, and communication in everyday activities. A functional approach to cognitive-communicative assessment would include measures at this level. As shown in Table 3-1, conversational or discourse skills, use of the telephone, and social skills are all considered at this level.

Handicap (or disability) is "a disadvantage for a given individual that limits or prevents the fulfillment of a role that is normal (depending on age,

Table 3-1. Classifications of effects of injury on the individual and examples.

WHO[a]	Nagi[b]	Examples
Impairment	Impairment	Reduced auditory comprehension Anomia Slowed information processing
Disability	Functional limitation	Reduced social skills Limited conversational skills Difficulty using telephone
Handicap	Disability	Inability to work, go to school Lack of meaningful relationships

[a] World Health Organization (1980)

[b] Nagi (1969)

sex, and social and cultural factors) for that individual" (WHO, 1980, p. 183). Examples of handicaps would include difficulty resuming a role as a parent, spouse, student, or employee due to brain injury. This level of assessment must consider relevant environmental factors that affect role resumption. Societal factors, such as attitudinal or structural barriers to role fulfillment, often contribute to a handicap. For example, a person with a head injury might be capable of returning to work but the individual's town lacks public transportation to the place of employment. Another individual might be capable of work, if the employer would provide a less distracting environment.

Three other considerations of outcomes after trauma are included by Whiteneck (1992). They are health, life satisfaction, and cost. *Health status* of an individual is important, because it affects a person's ability to fully participate and benefit from rehabilitation, as well as the individual's range of discharge options. An individual with serious ongoing medical issues, such as uncontrollable seizures or headaches or a fracture that will not heal, will experience rehabilitation program interruptions for treatment purposes and may even require intermittent rehospitalizations. Return to employment and independent living may be precluded by such medical complications.

Determination of an individual's perceived *life satisfaction* is also a consideration in evaluating the outcome of rehabilitation. This is often determined by simply asking an individual to self-rate quality of life or degree of satisfaction with his or her life (Whiteneck, 1992). More extensive questionnaires have been used to assess satisfaction within various life domains (Fugl-Meyer, Branholm, & Fugl-Meyer, 1991).

The *cost* of getting an individual to a certain outcome is another consideration. Responsible clinicians must be concerned about the efficiency of services provided and use cost and functional outcome information to evaluate their rehabilitation programs.

In summary, a complete cognitive-communication evaluation involves multiple steps to gather information concerning all aspects of an individual's life. The evaluator must consider all levels of outcome determination when devising an evaluation protocol and selecting methodologies. More specifically, the domains of knowledge to be assessed and possible methods to collect this data are outlined in Table 3-2. Using the road map developed in the previous chapters, the evaluation journey of hypothesis testing and discovery displayed in this table will be described in this chapter.

The First Step: Review of Pertinent Records

The first step in the evaluation process is to obtain and review records concerning the individual to be evaluated. These records generally include a written application or questionnaire completed by the individual or a family member prior to the evaluation along with past school, medical, and rehabilitation records. As shown in Table 3-2, this step provides the examiner with a preliminary understanding of the reason for the referral or need for services at the particular point in time, the person's preinjury and postinjury functioning, and relevant medical and injury data.

Obtaining this information prior to the evaluation is extremely important for several reasons. It guides the selection of appropriate assessment procedures and the scheduling and pacing of the evaluation process. For example, an individual with limited endurance and tolerance for frustration may need to have short sessions spaced over several days. The review alerts the examiner to any special sensory, motor, or medical concerns such as cortical blindness or hearing loss that would influence test selection or behavioral observations. Having a clear idea of the concerns of the referral source or the individual permits the selection of tests or approaches that will thoroughly assess the areas of concern. Knowledge of past history allows the clinician to detect inconsistencies, potential conflicts, and areas requiring more direct clarification. If the individual has been evaluated by other professionals, the input from other disciplines can help provide a more complete picture of the individual.

The records review process forms the basis of a comprehensive case history. However, additional input from the individual and a family member or significant other at the time of evaluation must be obtained to ensure the completeness and accuracy of the case history. In many instances, medical records contain inconsistencies or errors. In acute settings, complete social, developmental, educational, and vocational histories often are not obtained due to the emphasis on medical issues, limited time with the individual, or lack of a reliable source for this information.

Table 3–2. Domains and methodology for evaluation of functional communication.

	Reason for Referral	Premorbid Status	Injury and Health Issues	Cognitive-Communication Impairments	Functional Communication Abilities	Environmental Factors	Long-Term Goals
Review of records	X	X	X				
Interview of individual	X	X	X	X	X	X	X
Interview of family and/or significant others	X	X	X	X	X	X	X
Behavioral observations				X	X	X	
Formal, standardized testing				X			
Nonstandardized testing					X		
Needs assessment/Futures planning						X	X

Step Two: Interview of Individual and Family

Interviews of the individual and at least one significant other—spouse, parent, friend, or relative—provide critical information needed for several purposes in the evaluation process. One purpose of the interviews is to verify, clarify, and expand the information obtained in the record review. Use of the first three methods shown on Table 3-2—review of records, interview of person, and interview of family/significant other—to accumulate data on the presenting problem, preinjury functioning, injury-related information, and current health status constitutes a comprehensive case history.

A Comprehensive Case History

A comprehensive case history is extremely important for this population because of the heterogeneity of individual consequences. In addition, a case history helps to determine the effects of possible frontal lobe damage. There is wide variation in what is considered socially acceptable behavior among noninjured individuals; therefore, it is important to conduct a thorough investigation of premorbid behavior and of an individual's cultural and social influences and life experiences to detect any changes attributable to the injury (Hart & Jacobs, 1993).

A thorough review of events in an individual's life prior to the point of evaluation always has been important, but is even more critical when the overriding consideration is functional abilities. By understanding how an individual functioned to the point of evaluation and what happened in the individual's life to get the person to his or her current level, the examiner obtains not only a more holistic picture of the individual but also clues as to the origin of any cognitive and communication barriers.

As discussed in Chapter 1, ineffective interpersonal communication is a frequent sequela of brain injury. One must not make the mistake, however, of ignoring premorbid characteristics and abilities; many individuals with brain injury had preexisting problems with pyschosocial functioning or learning. Also, the majority of individuals with traumatic brain injury are adolescents or young adults, injured at a point in life when the development of adult social skills and social maturity, in all likelihood, was incomplete. In addition, because wide individual differences in psychosocial and communication functioning exist among noninjured individuals, premorbid communication style and interpersonal relationships should be investigated. Finally, postinjury influences on communication abilities, such as the lack of opportunity to learn or practice appropriate social skills due to nonnormalizing environments (e.g., a nursing home placement), poor adjustment to disability, or lack of appropriate rehabilitation can be uncovered by reviewing the records.

A former outpatient, Bob, provides an example of the importance of considering an individual's background and social environment. Bob talked excessively, cracked jokes with the receptionist and anyone walking by, and flirted with all the females, including his therapist. His overly friendly behavior was considered odd in a rehabilitation setting, but judgments about appropriateness had to be tempered by an understanding of his past and current life experiences. He was a 30-year-old confirmed bachelor who loved to gamble and socialize. After high school he had owned and operated a series of small businesses in a small town. At age 28 when he went bankrupt, he decided to become a casino dealer on a cruise ship, so he could get paid for spending his time gambling and socializing. He received his brain injury from a moped accident in Mexico, but had returned to work full-time by 9 months postinjury when evaluated by this author. His work friends and supervisor saw nothing unusual in his social behavior, only minor problems in his speed of calculation of payoffs and in dealing with obnoxious casino players. Intervention efforts, therefore, were not wasted on trying to change a premorbid behavior pattern that was appropriate for his environment.

The specific categories of information to be gleamed in a case history are listed in Table 3–3. A sample form for gathering case history information is given in Appendix A. Each category is critical to obtaining a holistic view of an individual and should be thoroughly investigated.

Medical History

The need for a thorough medical history cannot be overstated with this population. Information related to the brain injury and to current medical/health status provides insight into potential concerns in rehabilitation and the prognosis for additional recovery.

Presenting Problem. A good starting point is to obtain the views of an individual and family on the presenting problem or the initial circum-

Table 3-3. Categories of case history information.

Medical history

Developmental/Educational history

Psychosocial history

Work history

Leisure interests and activities

Communication/Personal style

Financial and legal issues

Transportation

stances of the brain injury, as well as the reason for seeking services at the present time of evaluation. For example, knowing that Amanda's father had been killed in the accident in which she was injured and that she had been driving at the time alerts the clinician that there may be significant family and personal adjustment issues requiring intervention.

Age. The age at which a person was injured should be specifically noted. This information suggests the level of the individual's premorbid social communication skill. In addition, age has been shown to be a determining factor of both return to work (Brooks et al., 1987) and postinjury living arrangement (Vogenthaler, Smith, & Goldfader, 1989).

Severity of Injury. Information related to the severity of the initial brain injury should be obtained:

1. Initial Glascow Coma Scale (GCS) (Teasdale & Jennett, 1974) score, especially the best GCS in the first 24 hours postinjury.
2. Length of coma.
3. Length of posttraumatic amnesia.
4. Pattern of CT or MRI findings.
5. Oculovestibular response.
6. Secondary intracranial complications such as hematomas, anoxia, or increased intracranial pressure.

Each of these has consistently been found to be a major predictor of long-term outcome (Alexandre, Colombo, Nertempi, & Benedetti, 1983; Eisenberg & Weiner, 1987).

Motor and Sensory Deficits. Knowledge of the motor and sensory deficits that remain from the injury alert you to adjustments that might be needed in assessment or treatment. For example, visual deficits, especially diplopia (double vision), are common after brain injury and will influence reading and spatial abilities and long-term academic or vocational needs and goals. The loss of smell also is found in a number of individuals with TBI, because of the location of the olfactory nerves on the inferior, orbital aspect of the frontal lobes. Anosmia, or the loss of the sense of smell, poses a safety hazard, as an individual is unable to smell fire or leaking gas. Affected individuals generally experience a loss in the sense of taste and may loose interest in food as a result. Anosmia has been associated with poor psychosocial and vocational outcomes (Martzke, Swan, & Varney, 1991).

Cognitive-Communicative Changes. The major changes in cognition, communication, and behavior as judged by the individual and family should be noted. More in-depth interview techniques to uncover these changes will be addressed later in this section.

Medications. Medication status is crucial because of the possible influences on cognitive and communication abilities. Certain medications, such as Valium® and Haldol®, may significantly reduce arousal and/or cognitive abilities (Zasler, 1991) and thereby influence test scores. Exploration of medication can lead to information about medical conditions or behavioral issues not included elsewhere. For example, no mention may be made about behavioral challenges until the clinician questions why the individual is taking certain medications. A list of medications, especially for neurobehavioral management, frequently prescribed for this population is found in Table 3–4. Additional information concerning pharmacological management after brain injury can be found in Blackerby and Gualtieri (1991), Gualtieri (1988), O'Shanick and Parmelee (1989), and Zasler (1991, 1992).

Medical Status. Medical status at time of assessment and ongoing medical problems are also important to note. The presence of a shunt or possible seizures signals the clinician to monitor fluctuations in cognitive and behavioral functioning. Often the clinician is the first to notice subtle changes resulting from a blocked shunt or medication toxicity, indicating a need for medical consultation.

Endocrine functioning and sleep patterns may be disturbed after brain injury and may require additional medical evaluation. There may be special dietary concerns, either due to preinjury conditions, such as high cholesterol, or caused by postinjury changes, such as dysphagia. In some instances, the individual may experience choking because of impulsive eating habits, despite adequate motor control of swallowing. Other individuals tend to overeat because they do not feel satiety or cannot self-monitor eating behavior.

Preinjury Medical History. Any significant preinjury injury, illness, or surgery should be listed. This is particularly important for individuals with a history of cardiovascular disease, polio, seizures, significant trauma, or other factors that would have affected premorbid physical and cognitive-communication abilities.

Rehabilitation History. A final aspect of the medical information to obtain is an account of what has happened to an individual from the point of injury to the time of evaluation. A person who has received intensive, specialized brain injury rehabilitation and yet not made progress may have little potential to benefit from additional services. However, someone who has not experienced an integrated rehabilitation program may have potential, even many years postinjury. By exploring the prior rate of recovery, the clinician can formulate an hypothesis regarding future progress.

Developmental/Educational History

The individual's childhood development of motor, speech, language, cognitive, and social abilities should be explored. Questions concerning a person's academic experiences are important as well. The highest level of education before the injury provides insight into premorbid academic skills and intellectual and learning capacity.

Table 3–4. Medications frequently prescribed and potential side effects.

Medication	Purpose	Side Effects
Psychostimulants		
Methylphenidate (Ritalin®)	Increase attention, concentration, and memory	Anorexia, insomnia, headache, irritability
Pemoline (Cylert®)	Elevate consciousness	Toxic effects: paranoid misinterpretations, hallucinations
Amphetamine (Dexedrine®)	Suppress fatigue, confusion	Addiction potential (Dexedrine)
Neurotransmitters		
Levodopa-carbidopa (Sinemet®)	Increase attention and initiation	Gastrointestinal upset, confusion, agitation
Bromocriptine (Parlodel®)	Elevate arousal	
Amantadine (Symmetrel®)	Treat agitation, aggression while recovering from coma	
	Treat side effects of neuroleptics	
Neuroleptics/Antipsychotics		
Haloperidol (Haldol®)	Control thought disorders	Tardive dyskinesia, tremor, acute dystonic reaction
Chlorpromazine (Thorazine®)	Decrease agitation, rage	Decreased attention and memory, sedation
Thioridazine (Mellaril®)	Decrease anxiety	Adverse effects on motor recovery
Clozapine (Clozaril®)		Lowered seizure threshold
Molindone (Moban®)		Neuroleptic malignant syndrome (unstable blood pressure and temperature, rigidity)
Antihypertensives		
(Beta-blockers)	Decrease blood pressure	Ventricular failure, bradycardia, hypotension, bronchial asthma, fatigue, sedation, depression, hallucinations
Propranolol (Inderal®)	Decrease agitation, rage	
Pindolol (Visken®)	Control headaches, essential tremors, anxiety	

Continued

Table 3–4. Continued

Medication	Purpose	Side Effects
Antispasticity		
Dantrolene sodium (Dantrium®)	Control spasticity, cramping of muscles, tightness	Liver toxicity, diarrhea
Baclofen (Lioresal®)		Dizziness, drowsiness, nausea
		Weakness
Antidepressants		
Tricyclics:	Treat depression, sleep disturbances	Anticholinergic symptoms (dry mouth, urinary retention, blurred vision, constipation)
Trazodone (Desyrel®)	May be used to decrease anxiety, agitation, confusion, headaches, emotional lability, aggressive behavior	
Imipramine (Tofranil®)		Rare: numbness and weakness of mouth
Desipramine (Norpramin®)		Fatigue, sedation, possible lowered seizure threshold
Amitriptyline (Elavil®)		
Nortriptyline (Pamelor®)		
Fluoxetine (Prozac®)		Limited anticholinergic, sedative, or cardiotoxic effects
Paroxetine (Paxil®)		Possible increased agitation
Monoamine-Oxidase Inhibitors:		Occasionally hypomanic symptoms, including pressured speech
Phenelzine (Nardil®)		Hypertensive crisis-requires patient to be on a tyramine-free diet (i.e., cheese, beers, wines)
Tranycypromine (Parnate®)		
Isocarboxazid (Marplan®)		
Antianxiety Agents		
Benzodiazepines	Relieve anxiety and tension	Dizziness and lightheadedness
Alprazolam (Xanax®)	Control rage and violent behavior	Anticholinergic symptoms
Lorazepam (Ativan®)	Relax muscles, control spasticity	Decreased cognitive functioning

Drug	Purpose	Side Effects
Diazepam (Valium®) Clorazepate (Tranxene®) Flurazepam (Dalmane®) Chlordiazepoxide (Librium®)	Dalmane: sleep disturbances	Paradoxical hostility, speech hesitations Interference with recovery and learning Adduction potential
Buspirone (BuSpar®)	Relieve anxiety Control behavioral disturbances Augment effect of lithium, carbamazepine, or valproic acid	Increased agitation, restlessness, racing thoughts, sedation
Lithium Carbonate (Lithobid®, Eskalith®)	Stabilize mood Treatment of bipolar disorder, rage, violent behavior, mania Improve lability, impulsivity	Confusion, slurred speech, sedation, unsteady gait, tremor Increased hostility Lowered seizure threshold Nausea, vomiting, diarrhea, anorexia
Anticonvulsants Carbamazepine (Tegretol®)	Prevent seizures Control rage or violent behavior Control secondary mania bipolar disorder, depression, or psychosis	Sensitivity to sunlight, nausea, liver abnormalities Dizziness, clumsiness, lightheadedness Dryness of mouth, sedation Ataxia Irritability
Clonazepam (Klonopin®)	Control seizures	Clumsiness or unsteadiness, dizziness, lightheadedness, drowsiness

Continued

Table 3–4. *Continued*

Medication	Purpose	Side Effects
Phenytoin (Dilantin®)	Control seizures	Tenderness, swelling or bleeding of the gums Unusual or excessive hair growth in young females Drowsiness, decreased concentration, dizziness Constipation, nausea and vomiting Ataxia when at toxic levels Decreased cognitive abilities Aggressive behavior, restlessness
Phenobarbital	Control seizures	Clumsiness and unsteadiness, ataxia, slurred speech Dizziness, drowsiness Decreased concentration and memory Lightheadedness Increased disinhibition and activity
Primidone (Mysoline®)	Control seizures	Sedation Increased disinhibition
Valproic acid (Depakene®) Divalproex sodium (Depakote®)	Control seizures, mania, rage	Stomach irritation, stomach or abdominal cramps, diarrhea Trembling of hands and arms, weight gain Interference with testing for diabetics, hepatoxicity Agitation

Premorbid learning problems also should be explored because of the frequency of occurrence in this population. Forty-four percent of persons admitted to an acute brain injury rehabilitation program have been found to have preinjury learning problems (Haas et al., 1987). This presents a number of implications for treatment and prognosis. For a person with a premorbid learning disability, a blow to the head no doubt will increase future risks and exacerbate the constellation of symptoms typically associated with learning disabilities: distractibility, short attention span, poor frustration tolerance, and inefficient information processing. The individual and significant other also can provide insight into premorbid learning style and study habits, areas particularly critical for those individuals wanting to return to school.

Psychosocial History

The influence of premorbid psychosocial functioning on postinjury behavior cannot be overstated. As reported in Chapter 1, premorbid psychopathology, including substance abuse, maladaptive interpersonal relationships, or psychiatric disturbances, is a relatively common finding in this population. Specific inquiries should be made concerning pre- and postinjury use of drugs or alcohol or psychiatric diagnoses. These are negative prognostic indicators and have implications for rehabilitation needs. Many times, the individual and significant others fail to spontaneously mention these aspects of the individual's life.

The use of tobacco also should be explored. Persons who smoke may need counseling about safety and health issues, especially when respiratory functioning or physical endurance are compromised by the injury. Use of smokeless tobacco can be life-threatening for individuals who aspirate liquids.

Family relationships and support networks are key aspects of psychosocial functioning. Clinical experience as well as research indicate that an individual's recovery and long-term psychosocial and vocational success are often dependent on family cohesion and social support (Barry & Clark, 1992; Kaplan, 1991). Information should be obtained about the individual's ability to develop and maintain friends and the current marital status. The occupation, marital status, educational background, and level of support of each family member is of relevance to the functioning of an individual.

Individual and family adjustment issues are another area to be discussed. Secondary reactions to the injury itself, such as depression and increased frustration, are likely at the postacute stage of rehabilitation, as the individual begins to face the long-term consequences of brain injury and adjusts personal goals, expectations, and aspirations (Fordyce, Roueche, & Prigatano, 1983). The adjustment of the family and acceptance of realistic rehabilitation goals are critical. Overprotective parents may keep an individual from achieving the highest level of functioning possible; whereas overzealous parents may keep moving the individual from program to program. If an individual is married, the marital relationship should be explored. Spouses may want to end the marriage, but have problems dealing with this. Questions about these issues can identify the need for a referral for counseling.

Cultural, social, and religious factors that might influence the rehabilitation program should be explored with the family and the individual. Cultural beliefs about medical care and disability may cause distrust and lack of acceptance of a team's recommendations.

Work History

Accurate work information is not always easy to obtain for an adult client, because an individual can often be a poor informant and the parents may be unfamiliar with their adult offspring's work history. Knowing a person's occupation, however, reveals the cognitive and communication tasks that a person performed prior to the injury. It gives insight into premorbid intellectual abilities and possible preserved skills and abilities. In addition, if the individual experienced difficulty maintaining employment preinjury, the examiner should suspect problems with interpersonal relationships, substance abuse, and/or psychiatric problems.

For example, Rick was never able to keep a job longer than 6 months before he was injured, frequently blowing up at his boss or co-workers when he was treated "unjustly." His injury made his coping and anger management skills and rigid thinking even worse. Prognosis for a favorable outcome, especially as the funding source was the state department of vocational rehabilitation, was guarded. Treatment had to immediately and aggressively address these issues.

Information that might be helpful regarding future job placement also should be gathered. Communication with the last place of employment is critical when there is any possibility for return to that company. Family resources are also important when considering return to work. Often when there is a family business, special adaptations can be made, or positions created to suit the needs of the person injured. With sufficient financial resources, an individual with even a severe brain injury can be assisted in starting a business.

Leisure Interests and Activities

Hobbies, social activities, community involvement in religious or civic organizations and volunteer activities, and other leisure interests and activities, both pre and post-injury, should be explored in taking a complete case history. Again, knowledge of a person's cognitive abilities and possible preserved skills and aptitudes can be gained. In addition, it alerts the clinician to topics and activities that interest and motivate an individual. For example, one young man with reduced reading comprehension had a strong interest in cars. Car magazines sparked his interest in learning to read better. Another young man enjoyed playing darts. He was rewarded for achieving weekly goals with planned outings to a local cafe/tavern hosting dart tournaments.

Communication/Personal Style

The person's primary language is an obvious consideration prior to the evaluation. When the focus is on functional abilities, it is also important to understand the premorbid communication style. This provides information on previous linguistic, executive, and social abilities.

An example is a 30-year-old single woman who had lived in the country and worked by herself in a small office all of her life until her injury. By family and self-report, she was a quiet, introverted person. Her postinjury behavior was characterized by poor initiation, planning, sequencing, and tolerance for feedback. She was anxious at being placed in group activities because of the physical closeness and communication involved. She disliked any structure placed on her and having to participate in group leisure activities in the community. Even all-day interaction with others, especially persons placing demands on her, as is typical in a rehabilitation program, was hard for her to tolerate. The interaction of her premorbid interactional style with frontal lobe damage resulted in lack of success in a rehabilitation facility.

Financial and Legal Issues

Funding. It is important that the clinician explore the financial resources at the disposal of an individual. Knowledge of the funding source for rehabilitation is critical, because the constraints of that funding source may influence clinical management and procedures. Medical insurance companies generally want documentation in traditional medical terms, specifying diagnosis and deficit areas, treatment plans that indicate medical necessity (especially safety and life-preserving issues and independent living functioning), and progress reports detailing discrete skills.

Vocational rehabilitation agencies, on the other hand, often do not want complex medical terminology. The vocational counselor instead needs information about the vocational implications of the deficits and how treatment will assist the individual in obtaining and maintaining employment. A third source of reimbursement, Medicare, places emphasis on functional abilities and functional communication goals.

Knowledge of financial resources also allows the clinician to determine if referral to community resources or governmental social agencies is needed, as when a person might qualify for Medicaid or Medicare benefits. Conservation of funds is an important ethical issue for all health care workers. They must be cognizant of the lifelong needs of individuals and make efforts to conserve funds to meet these needs.

Financial Disincentives. The presence of financial disincentives for returning to work or completing rehabilitation is another consideration. These disincentives include large disability income and litigation. If the individual draws a substantial disability income, there is little incentive to strive for returning to work. Clear and honest appraisal of abilities and long-term goal setting often are not possible if a lawsuit is in progress. Clinicians must operate somewhat cautiously in these cases, because motivation for seeking professional opinion or treatment may not be made clear at first. Settlements are often a mixed blessing. Although a settlement can provide financial resources for obtaining appropriate rehabilitation services, some individuals become miraculously "cured" when the settlement is obtained.

Criminal/Legal Activity. Inquiry should be made regarding previous arrests, outstanding warrants, or probation or investigations into criminal activity. These are all negative factors for potential to benefit from rehabilitation.

Guardianship. A final issue is guardianship. It is often in individuals' best interest to have their own guardianship, so they feel empowered to make decisions and control their own lives. Family members who obtained guardianship at an earlier stage of recovery, however, may not be willing to give up this power, even when the rehabilitation team feels they should, because of a "need" to have the individual dependent on them, a fear of letting go of control, or a self-serving desire to control the money. In other cases, when poor judgment is displayed by the individual, a guardian or conservator may be needed to assist in the management of money and making major life decisions. This is particularly true when there is a legal settlement that must be conserved for lifelong needs and the individual lacks a long-range perspective on spending.

Transportation

Access to transportation may be a crucial factor in the individual being able to attend treatment on a regular basis or returning to work in a desired location after rehabilitation. A driving evaluation is important before an individual attempts to return to operating a vehicle. Knowing the types of transportation available in the discharge community assists in setting appropriate long-term goals.

Assessment of Past and Current Functioning

Another purpose of interviewing the individual and a significant other is to obtain the perspectives of each person regarding past and current cognitive-communication functioning, especially in functional activities. The individual and the significant other are the ones most familiar with the level of preinjury functioning and events since the injury. Because the family or significant other generally has had a chance to observe the individual across a range of natural settings by the time the individual is at the postacute stage, valuable insights can be provided concerning cognitive, language, emotional, behavioral, and executive functioning in real-life situations.

Areas that should be explored during the interview process include:

1. Individual and family perceptions of the individual's strengths and needs at the current time.
2. Long-term goals for the individual.
3. Expectations the family and individual have of the clinician or rehabilitation program.
4. A typical day for the individual.

By interviewing the individual and family member at the same time, the clinician can determine any discrepancies between the client's view of his or her abilities and the family's views. Insight is gained into the individual's self-awareness, relationships within the family unit, and how each person handles feedback and disagreement (Prigatano, Pepping, & Klonoff, 1986). The use of interviews will be covered under other sections of this chapter, as appropriate.

Specific interview questionnaires have been developed to use with the family or with the individual. Levin, High et al. (1987) developed the Neurobehavioral Rating Scale in response to the need to characterize the behavioral changes after brain injury. Ratings are determined by the clinician based on an interview and mental status examination. This scale has been found sensitive to frontal lobe symptomotology. The General Health and History Questionnaire was developed by Kreutzer and colleagues (Kreutzer, Leininger, Doherty, & Waaland, 1987; Kreutzer & Wehman, 1990) to gather information on somatic, cognitive, social/communication, and behavioral functioning. The Iowa Collateral Head Injury Interview (Varney, 1991; Varney & Menefee, 1993) is an interview protocol designed to elicit information about changes in psychosocial functioning after TBI. Varney and Menefee (1993) point out that persons familiar with the individual, such as parents, spouse, siblings, and co-workers, can identify changes in cognitive, social, behavioral, and interpersonal functioning that cannot be reliably assessed through standardized testing nor through self-report.

Step Three: Behavioral Observations

Keen observational skills are particularly important in dealing with the population with TBI because of the need to assess functional abilities and frontal lobe dysfunction—both elusive with standardized testing. As shown in Table 3–2, the purpose of the observations is to gather information regarding cognitive-communicative impairments, functional communication abilities, and environmental influences on communication.

Observation begins with the very first interaction with an individual in the waiting room and continues through the formal standardized testing, ending only when involvement with the individual is terminated. Observations foster the generation and testing of hypotheses about communicative competence. To obtain a complete sample of behaviors, observations should be made in a variety of settings and activities and with a variety of partners (Sbordone, 1991).

Observations made during standardized testing procedures form the backbone of the "process" approach to neuropsychological testing (Kaplan, 1988). In this approach, qualitative information is accumulated regarding *how* the individual arrives at answers on a standardized test, not just whether the responses were right or wrong. The individual's approach to a task and style of interaction with the clinician are noted, as well as the ability to adapt and cope with the demands of evaluation procedures.

Recording Observational Data

These general behavioral observations should be recorded in a systematic manner. One way is through use of a checklist, such as the one in Appendix B. This form permits the recording of general observations about aspects of attention, memory, executive functions/metacognition, response style, affect, and motivation.

Attention

The ability of an individual to maintain and shift attention across the assessment procedures can be noted. Observations can answer the following types of questions.

Does arousal or alertness vary over time?

Is the individual able to maintain attention to each task until it is completed or are reminders needed?

Is the individual able to shift to a new task as required?

Is the individual able to inhibit response to extraneous objects, noises, or stimuli in the environment?

Is the individual able to process instructions at a normal rate or does the examiner have to reduce the rate?

Does the individual demonstrate difficulty maintaining attention over time due to fatigue?

Memory

Observations can reveal the adequacy of memory processes as well.

Does the individual require repetition of instructions or need steps to be broken into smaller units?

Does the individual confabulate when memory failures are present?

Does the individual attempt to reauditorize or repeat information to process it?

Does the individual repeat his or her previous statements or topics in conversation?

Does the individual perform better in cued rather than free recall?

Executive/Metacognitive Functioning

Information can be gained about the individual's executive functions or metacognitive abilities from observations during testing.

Does the individual demonstrate awareness and concern for his or her level of performance?

Does the individual use strategies to improve performance?

Is he or she aware of the use of strategies?

Does the individual monitor and adjust the strategy to the task?

Individuals can be asked to "think aloud" as they perform a task, enabling the clinician to monitor their thought processes (Cicerone & Tupper, 1986).

Response Patterns

The quality and control of responding should also be observed.

Does the individual demonstrate problems in fine motor control or motor slowing?

Is the individual impulsive, responding before directions are completed?

Does the individual keep repeating a particular response or perseverate on a task?

Does the individual engage in nonpurposeful movements, such as utilization behavior (nonpurposeful use of objects in the environment, such as a pencil, when not appropriate)?

Affect

Observations can also reveal aspects of emotional functioning.

Does the individual appear overly anxious by inquiring about performance or making disparaging remarks?

Does the individual demonstrate immature responses or remarks?

Is anger or frustration displayed?

Is there a range of emotions that are displayed?

Drive/Motivation

Finally, judgments can be made as to overall drive and motivation.

Does the individual display an appropriate level of effort?

Does the individual initiate any questions or conversation on his or her own?

Is the individual generally cooperative and compliant with instructions and demands?

In addition to these general behavioral observations, more specific observational techniques are important in assessing functional communication abilities and environmental needs. These will be discussed under those headings.

Step Four: Standardized Testing of Component Processes

The evaluation of component processes is conducted to identify and describe the impairments in cognitive, linguistic, and executive functioning that influence and limit functional communication skills following TBI. Because performance can be compared with established norms, areas of significantly decreased functioning can be determined. Standardization of scores permits the detection of intraindividual variation across areas or processing strengths and weaknesses that will influence all areas of real-life functioning. With this knowledge, the clinician can assist an individual in developing compensatory strategies to use across functional settings, in developing treatment to improve the areas of need, in identifying realistic long-term goals, and in capitalizing on strengths.

As shown in Table 3–2, interviews, observations, and standardized testing are used in an integrated manner to identify and describe the impairments in cognitive, linguistic, psychosocial, and executive functioning that contribute to an individual's social communication performance. Although problems exist in the ecological validity of traditional cognitive and linguistic testing approaches when used in isolation, these procedures still serve a vital role in the evaluation process. By incorporating behavioral observations, as mentioned in the previous section, the informational capacity of standardized testing is increased. Testing the limits, or continuing of testing beyond standard time limits, also can be used to determine capability without time restriction.

Because language, cognitive, and executive skills are so interwoven, an evaluation of language should be conducted as part of a complete neuropsychological evaluation. In a rehabilitation setting, a complete neuropsychological evaluation is generally conducted as a team evaluation, with input from several disciplines. The components of cognitive-linguistic functioning evaluated include orientation, attention, learning and memory, visuospatial perception and integration, language, sensory and motor functions, abstract reasoning/judgment, intellectual functioning, and executive functioning. A personality assessment is also an important part of a complete neuropsychological evaluation (Prigatano et al., 1986).

As a general rule, each rehabilitation team selects standardized tests from a flexible battery based on the needs of the facility and persons served and divides responsibilities for coverage of all areas. Kreutzer, Leininger, and Harris (1990) and Sohlberg and Mateer (1989a) suggest the following guidelines when selecting appropriate tests to include in the neuropsychological battery from among the diverse tests available:

1. Tests with proven reliability and validity.
2. Tests typically used with adults with brain injuries.
3. Tests that assess aspects of cognitive functioning as discretely as possible.
4. Multiple tests of each cognitive domain.
5. Tests with adequate normative data.
6. Tests with relevance to real-life functioning.

Table 3–5 lists standardized tests that have been identified as useful in tapping each aspect of cognitive and executive functioning after TBI. Excellent guidelines for the selection and interpretation of standardized neuropsychological testing can be found in Baxter, Cohen, and Ylvisaker (1985); Kreutzer, Devany, Myers, and Marwitz (1991); Kreutzer et al. (1990); Lezak (1983, 1989, 1993); Prigatano et al. (1986); Sohlberg and Mateer (1989a; 1989b); and Spreen and Strauss (1991) and, therefore, are not reviewed here.

Standardized testing of linguistic abilities at the postacute stage is not a simple process. No single test exists that meets the needs of individuals who do not have aphasia, with recovery to Level VII and above on the Rancho Los Amigos Levels of Cognitive Functioning (Hagen, 1984; Hagen & Malkmus, 1979). Due to the range of impairments and more subtle nature of possible linguistic deficits, many clinicians find that the best approach is to select aphasia battery subtests that tap the desired areas and to supplement these results with other standardized tests of language

Table 3-5.   Standardized neuropsychological tests.

Attention

Sustained attention   Digit Span—*Wechsler Memory Scale-Revised* (WMS-R)
(Wechsler, 1987); or *Wechsler Adult Intelligence Scale-Revised* (WAIS-R) (Wechsler, 1981)
Seashore Rhythm Test (Reitan & Wolfson, 1985)

Selective attention   *Stroop Color and Word Test* (Golden, 1978; Stroop, 1935)
Trail Making Test (Reitan, 1958; Reitan & Wolfson, 1985)
Letter Cancellation Task (Ponsford & Kinsella, 1992)

Processing speed   Simple and Four Choice Reaction Time (Van Zomeren,
1981)
Paced Auditory Serial Addition Test (PASAT) (Gronwall, 1977;
Gronwall & Sampson, 1974)
Symbol Digit Modalities Test (Smith, 1973)

Memory

Verbal   Selective Reminding Test (Buschke & Fuld, 1974; Hannay
& Levin, 1985)
California Verbal Learning Test (Delis, Kramer, Kaplan, &
Ober, 1986)
Auditory-Verbal Learning Test (Rey, 1964)

Visual   *The Revised Visual Retention Test* (Benton, 1974)
Recognition Memory Test (Warrington, 1984)
Rey-Osterreith Complex Figure—Immediate and Delayed
Recall (Lezak, 1983; Rey, 1941)

Verbal and Visual   WMS-R (Wechsler, 1987)

Everyday tasks   *Rivermead Behavioural Memory Test* (Wilson, Cockburn, &
Baddeley, 1985)

**Visuospatial
 Perception and
 Construction**

Visuospatial
  Perception   *Benton Test of Facial Recognition* (Benton, Hamsher, Varney,
& Spreen, 1983)
Hooper Visual Organization Test (Hooper, 1958, 1983)

Visuoconstruction   Block Design from WAIS-R (Wechsler, 1981)
Rey-Osterreith Complex Figure Copy (Lezak, 1983; Rey,
1941; Spreen & Strauss, 1991)
Clock Drawing (Spreen & Strauss, 1991)

Motor   Finger Tapping Test (Reitan & Wolfson, 1985)

Intelligence   WAIS-R (Wechsler, 1981

**Executive
 Functioning**

Planning   Tower of London (Shallice, 1982; Shallice & Burgess,
1991)
Porteus Maze Test (Porteus, 1959, 1965)

	Rey-Osterreith Complex Figure-Copy (Lezak, 1983; Rey, 1941)
	Tinkertoy Test (Lezak, 1983, 1993)
Productivity & Self-regulation	*Ruff Figural Fluency Test* (D'Elia & Boon, 1993; Ruff, Light, & Evans, 1987)
	Design Fluency Test (Jones-Gotman & Milner, 1977)
	Controlled Oral Word Association Test from Multilingual Aphasia Examination (MAE) (Benton & Hamsher, 1983)
Concept formation and Flexibility of thinking	*Wisconsin Card Sorting Test* (Heaton, 1981)

functioning (Groher & Ochipa, 1992; Hartley, 1990; Kennedy & De-Ruyter, 1991; Milton & Wertz, 1986; Sohlberg & Mateer, 1989a; Ylvisaker & Holland, 1985). For some deficit areas there is no adequate standardized test for adults, so batteries designed for children or informal measures must be used. Table 3–6 lists standardized tests or informal measures that are frequently used to measure linguistic abilities.

The primary consideration, however, is to sample all modalities and levels of language processing in a hierarchical manner to establish processing strengths and needs and to determine an individual's learning style. At a minimum, the testing should evaluate:

1. Auditory and reading comprehension of single words, questions, directions, and paragraphs.
2. Verbal memory and learning, including orientation and recall of biographical information.
3. Oral expression of words (both naming of pictures and rapid word association), sentence generation, and picture description.
4. Written expression of words, sentences, and paragraphs; spelling; mechanics of writing (grammar, punctuation and capitalization), and legibility.
5. Verbal integration and semantic organization.
   a. Word meanings, associations, and categorization
   b. Sequencing of steps
   c. Comparison and contrast, analogies
   d. Scripts, story schemata
6. Abstract language, such as humor, proverbs, and idiomatic expressions.
7. Use of language for problem solving and reasoning.

Considerations When Testing

To conclude this section on standardized testing, several precautions need to be raised. One is that the clinician must always consider the effect of

Table 3–6.   Tests of linguistic processes.

Component Process	Applicable Tests/Subtests
Auditory Comprehension	
Spoken vocabulary	*Peabody Picture Vocabulary Test-Revised* (PPVT-R) (Dunn & Dunn, 1981)
Questions	*Minnesota Test for Differential Diagnosis of Aphasia* (MTDDA) (Schuell, 1972)—Understanding Sentences
	Wiig-Semel Test of Linguistic Concepts (Wiig & Semel, 1974)
Directions/ Commands	*Revised Token Test* (McNeil & Prescott, 1978)
	Boston Diagnostic Aphasia Examination (BDAE) (Goodglass & Kaplan, 1983)—Following Commands
	Neurosensory Center Comprehensive Examination for Aphasia-Revised (NCCEA) (Spreen & Benton, 1977)—Token Test
Paragraphs	BDAE (Goodglass & Kaplan, 1983) or MTDDA (Schuell, 1972)—Paragraph Comprehension
Verbal Memory/ Learning	
Attention/ Immediate recall	WMS-R (Wechsler, 1981)—Memory Span Subtest
Sentence repetition	*Western Aphasia Battery* (WAB) (Kertesz, 1982); BDAE—Sentence Repetition
Prose recall	WMS-R—Logical Memory (Immediate and Delayed Recall) (Wechsler, 1981)
Verbal learning	WMS-R (Wechsler, 1981)—Associate Learning (Wechsler, 1981); *California Verbal Learning Test* (Delis, Kramer, Kaplan, & Ober, 1986)
Orientation/ Personal information	*Ross Information Processing Assessment* (Ross, 1986); Galveston Orientation and Amnesia Test (GOAT) (Levin, O'Donnell, & Grossman, 1979)
Oral Expression	
Confrontation naming	*Boston Naming Test* (Kaplan, Goodglass, & Weintraub, 1983)
	WAB (Kertesz, 1982)—Object Naming; BDAE (Goodglass & Kaplan, 1983)—Picture Naming
Verbal fluency/ Rapid word association	*Multilingual Aphasia Examination* (MAE) (Benton & Hamsher, 1983)—Controlled Oral Word Association Test
	BDAE (Goodglass & Kaplan, 1983) or WAB (Kertesz, 1982)—Animal Naming
	NCCEA (Spreen & Benton, 1977)—Word Fluency
Answering questions	BDAE (Goodglass & Kaplan, 1983)—Responsive Naming

Component Process	Applicable Tests/Subtests
Sentence generation	MTDDA (Schuell, 1972)—Sentence Generation
Picture description	BDAE (Goodglass & Kaplan, 1983)—Cookie Theft Picture
	WAB (Kertesz, 1982)—Spontaneous Speech Content and Fluency Scales
Verbal Integration and Reasoning with Language	
Semantic knowledge	*The Word Test* (Jorgenson, Barrett, Huisingh, &
Word association	Zachman, 1981)
Comparison and	*Detroit Tests of Learning Aptitude* (Hammill, 1985)
contrast	MTDDA (Schuell, 1972)—Defining words
Categorization	*Woodcock-Johnson Psychoeducational Battery* (Woodcock &
Analogies	Johnson, 1977)
Word definitions	Informal tests
Multiple meanings of words	
Verbal absurdities	
Abstract language	
Humor	
Proverbs	
Idiomatic expressions	
Problem solving and reasoning	

Note: From "Assessment of Functional Communication" (p. 144) by L. L. Hartley, 1990. In D. Tupper and K. Cicerone (Eds.), *The Neuropsychology of Everyday Life. Vol. 1: Assessment and Basic Competencies.* Boston: Kluwer Academic. Copyright 1990 by Kluwer Academic Publishers. Adapted by permission.

sensory changes on test-taking performance. For example, diplopia (double vision) may interfere with the accurate perception of regular printed material. Hearing always should be screened. Total loss of hearing in one or both ears has been reported in 8% of individuals hospitalized with brain injuries (Howe & Miller, 1975). Many more have some degree of injury-related or preexisting hearing loss. Even a mild loss, especially when combined with attentional and processing speed problems, can result in significant difficulty in understanding conversation (Wenzinger, Nemec, DePompei, & Flexer, 1991).

A second precaution is that the accuracy and validity of test data can be influenced by a host of factors unrelated to the areas supposedly being measured. These include motivation to present a certain profile or to succeed, fatigue, medications, mood status (e.g., anxiety, depression), and cultural beliefs and differences (Sbordone, 1991). All of these need to be explored and considered in an analysis of results.

A third precaution is that performance on one measure of a certain cognitive or executive process does not always equate to an individual's actual capacity in that area and certainly does not equate to functional application of that process (Sbordone, 1991). The former is true because each cognitive process, such as attention, has multiple components and subskills. The latter is true because standardized tests cannot fully evaluate frontal lobe dysfunction. Clinicians must look for collaborating evidence through use of other methods of evaluation, such as functional measures and observations.

Step Five: Environmental Needs Assessment

The next step in the evaluation process is to conduct an environmental needs assessment, an analysis of the individual's social and physical environment. Another name for this is an ecological inventory (Falvey, 1989). The purposes are to determine the relevant contexts of communication for an individual, to identify activities that are relevant and important in an individual's life, and to explore the impact of the environment on the individual's cognitive-communicative abilities. In terms of levels of outcome as listed in Figure 3–1, this step not only identifies the disabilities or functional limitations caused by a brain injury, but also the resulting role limitations or handicaps.

This step is necessary because there is such wide variation in functional skills needed even by individuals who are deemed "normal." Cultural and social expectations determine the level of skills needed even for individuals who are nondisabled. For example, a male high-school dropout who holds a manual labor job and whose wife handles all family financial and household affairs will have different cognitive-communication needs than an unmarried graduate student who lives on her own in a metropolitan area. In certain cultures, some functional life activities such as housekeeping, laundry, or cooking are seen as women's work and are not, under any circumstances, to be conducted by a man.

An environmental needs assessment begins by identifying the present and future environments within the major life domains (Valletutti & Dummett, 1992). As shown in Table 3–7, life domains can be classified in several ways. The activities, roles, and communication partners that are a part of current environments within those domains, as well as those that will be a part of the projected long-term environments, are then identified through the needs assessment.

A systematic method for gathering, tracking, and compiling this data is necessary. Two different methods are provided in Appendixes C and D. The form in Appendix D permits a more detailed analysis of activities and

Table 3-7. Various classifications of life domains (read down in columns).

Life	Personal Adjustment and Relationships	Domestic Living
Work	Daily Living Activities	Community Living
Play	Vocational/Educational	Leisure
	Leisure	School
		Vocational/Avocational

skills. Competence in the performance of the activities also can be indicated on both types of inventories. The Functional Independence Measure (1–7 rating) from the Uniform Data System (Granger, Hamilton, & Kayton, 1986) can be used or some other coding of level of independence can be employed. Input for completing an Environmental Needs Inventory can come from interviews of the individual and family, from observations, or through a questionnaire.

The needs assessment helps to bridge the gap between therapy and real-life needs and to generate socially meaningful goals. It provides a mechanism for obtaining family and client input regarding personal and cultural values or priorities for rehabilitation. In addition, it guides the selection of appropriate contexts for observing the social communication of the individual for evaluation of functional abilities (see next section). Data from the needs assessment are compared with other assessment information to determine the discrepancies between current abilities or skills and the skills needed to function in the current environment. Therapeutic goals, content, and materials can be selected that will build skills needed in current settings and prepare the individual for the desired long-term outcomes.

The actual use of a needs assessment like the ones in Appendixes C and D may depend on the role of the speech-language pathologist with a given individual. In an interdisciplinary work setting, information for such an ecological inventory may be gathered during the evaluation process by a number of different disciplines, including social work, occupational therapy, case management, physical therapy, vocational rehabilitation, and education, as well as speech-language pathology. A solo provider may have the entire responsibility for such an inventory.

As previously discussed, the needs assessment is used in the assessment stage to identify contexts in which functional abilities should be evaluated. It is used in treatment planning to establish priorities and to set socially relevant cognitive-communication goals. The application of this information by speech-language pathologists in treatment may vary. In some settings, the speech-language pathologist may work directly on an identified functional activity, such as preparing a meal or riding the bus. In almost all situations, the speech-language pathologist will work on the communication skills that are directly involved in functional activities (e.g., asking for information over the phone, reading a bus schedule, interviewing for a job). Additional goals can be to develop compensatory strategies needed in the identified everyday activities and to build the communication skills necessary for the employment of these compensatory strategies (e.g., reading a schedule in his or her memory book or writing down errands). The needs assessment also guides the selection of therapy materials and topics of relevance to an individual's functional needs.

Step Six: Evaluation of Everyday Performance

The final step of the evaluation process is to evaluate an individual's actual cognitive-communicative performance in everyday activities. This step focuses on communication ability at the disability or functional limitation level (see Figure 3–1) by examining how an individual with TBI communicates in everyday situations. The emphasis is on assessing functional, integrative behaviors that require the coordination of the component skills and systems assessed through standardized procedures (Szekeres et al., 1985).

Methodological Considerations

As stated in previous chapters, the difficulty at this level is that there is no consensus regarding the essential components of functional communication and how best to assess communicative competence. Literature from the areas of behavioral assessment, interpersonal competence, and pragmatics within speech-language pathology suggests several methodological considerations.

Level of Specificity

One consideration is the *level of specificity of judgments of social behaviors* on a continuum from molar to molecular. Global, or molar, procedures are usually either ratings of overall, subjective characteristics of social performance or checklists of items to be observed (Farrell, Rabinowitz, Wallender, & Curran, 1985; Prutting & Kirchner, 1983, 1987; Spitzberg & Hurt, 1987). Molar recordings are helpful in summarizing complex judgments of the effectiveness of an individual's communication, but, if too broad, do not provide the detail needed for treatment planning.

Molecular techniques, on the other extreme, involve more direct recordings (e.g., frequency, duration) of discrete, specific communication behaviors (e.g., eye gaze, talk time, utterances spoken). Molecular measures are more objective and provide information regarding specific behaviors of the individual in a specific situation. Criticisms of these procedures center on their unproven relationship to overall social competence (Conger et al., 1989) and the length of time required for analysis (Bedrosian, 1985).

Selection of Direct Versus Indirect Methods

Another consideration in assessing functional performance is *choice of indirect or direct methods* of data collection. Indirect methods include interviews, self-report, or ratings by others familiar with the individual (Nelson & Hayes, 1981). Direct methods of data collection include measurements taken by the clinician. These include:

1. Observation of communication events over a variety of natural settings.
2. Observation of unstructured social interactions in a clinical setting, preferably videotaped for later analysis.
3. Analysis of behaviors while engaged in simulation or role-playing of real-life events.
4. Quantitative measures of discourse comprehension and production.

No one method provides a complete picture of an individual's communication competence. The best strategy is to combine approaches that suit the needs of an individual, the purpose of the evaluation, and the constraints of the clinician's work environment.

Ethnographic Techniques

Another relevant body of literature is ethnography and its application to the study of communication (Crago & Cole, 1991; Ripich & Spinelli, 1985). Ethnographic techniques have been used by anthropologists and sociolinguists to study events and interactions to ascertain the underlying structure and rules of a particular culture (e.g., Native American tribes, courtroom discourse, classroom discourse). The field of pragmatics expanded the window of understanding communication disorders by emphasizing the need to consider how language is used within natural settings. Ethnography broadens the window even further by placing a stronger emphasis on the sociocultural context of the use of language and the need to examine local systems of knowledge and social structure (Crago & Cole, 1991).

Ethnographic assessment involves obtaining multiple input from interviews and observations to describe the behavior of the individual in multiple life experiences, to make inferences about the origins of that behavior, and to identify the salient aspects of any communication difficulties (Ripich & Spinelli, 1985). The evaluator arrives without preconceived notions and uses inductive reasoning to analyze the interview and observational data and identify communication strengths and needs.

Ethnographic research also has pointed out the need to consider cultural differences not only in terms of explaining the individual's performance, but also biases in the clinician's perceptions. Crago and Cole (1991) list various dimensions of social interactions that may vary across cultures. These include the mode of communication, the amount of talk, topics of discussion, dominance of communication partners, turn taking, speech acts, the role of language in the culture, and male-female communication patterns. Cole (1989) presents a chart of differences in communication norms across cultures. For example, avoidance of direct eye contact is considered by certain Hispanic and Native American cultures to be a sign of respect and attentiveness, whereas other cultures might consider it to be a lack of attentiveness and respect. Rehabilitation professionals must be sensitive to their own cultural standards and biases when evaluating someone from another culture. In addition, cultural variations in perceptions of persons with disabilities and trust in the value of Western medical practices may influence the rehabilitation of an individual.

Although listening and speaking are intrinsically related to one another in social communication, they will be discussed separately to outline techniques that emphasize one over the other. Methods that assess interactional behavior will be addressed under the speaking section.

Assessing Everyday Listening Skills

The Importance of Listening Skills

Listening is the most frequently used communication skill. Approximately 55% of adult verbal communication time is spent listening, as compared with 23% for speaking, 13% for reading, and 8% for writing. Workers spend an average of 60% of their work day listening (Brown, 1982).

Listening is also the most important functional communication skill; appropriate interpersonal communication is predicated on the ability to understand the other person's message. Good listening skills are also necessary tools for problem solving, learning, and social growth. Listening is the communication skill that is most important for job success (DiSalvo & Steere, 1980), for career competence (Painter, 1985), and for entry level positions (Murphy & Jenks, 1982).

Development of Listening Ability

The natural development of listening skill occurs through the acquisition of skills and knowledge. Comprehension of words and ideas improves as concepts and schemata are acquired. The ways that schemata facilitate comprehension were discussed in Chapter 2. Language skill development in terms of phonemic discrimination and syntactic and semantic processing is another factor in the acquisition of comprehension abilities in children. A third factor is the development of skills and strategies for the overall semantic structure, theme development, and discourse organization. A later development is the ability to determine comprehension breakdowns and inconsistencies. A final factor is the development of the intent to understand and commitment to social interaction. This involves understanding of the social obligation to make sure that comprehension is accurate and the need for willful intent to listen actively.

Identification of Listening Skills

Despite the importance of listening skills and the likelihood of problems in this area after brain injury (see Chapter 2), clinicians often devote only limited attention to evaluating functional listening skills. This is no doubt because there are few standardized tests of comprehension for adults beyond the sentence level and few sources of information on functional listening skills. The *Boston Diagnostic Aphasia Examination* (Goodglass & Kaplan, 1983) contains a listening section of four paragraphs of varying lengths, discourse type, and abstractness. However, the types of questions asked are limited and the content unfamiliar to many young adults. The paragraph in the *Minnesota Test for Differential Diagnosis of Aphasia* (Schuell, 1972) is long and complex. Other approaches must be developed to best assess functional listening.

Guidelines on everyday listening skills can be found in Backlund, Brown, Gurry, and Jandt (1982); Boyce and Larson (1983); Lundsteen (1979); Schwartz and McKinley (1984); and Vallettuti and Dummett (1992). Publications of the Speech Communication Association also provide guidance (See Appendix M for address). Listening skills felt to be crucial to everyday functioning, synthesized from these resources, are listed in Table 3–8.

Literal comprehension has to do with obtaining factual information such as a main idea and its supporting details as well as a sequence of ideas. This is the type of comprehension needed to follow most directions. Interpretive or inferential comprehension involves going beyond what is explicitly stated to make inferences, to draw conclusions, to make predictions, to summarize, and to make comparisons of ideas. Critical listening involves the making of value judgments regarding the information, such as detecting the speaker's purpose, validity, motivation, and appropriateness. Metacognitive aspects involve the monitoring and correcting of communicative breakdowns.

Factors That Influence Listening

The ability to employ the above listening skills in everyday situations, however, may vary due to a number of different factors. As mentioned in

Table 3-8.   Taxonomy of listening skills.

Literal Level
  Detecting and remembering main ideas
  Identifying supporting details
  Identifying sequence or organization
  Paraphrasing
  Following spoken directions

Interpretive Level
  Making inferences, drawing conclusions
  Summarizing
  Interpreting abstract ideas and language
  Making generalizations
  Comparing and contrasting

Critical Level
  Discriminating relevant versus irrelevant information
  Detecting speaker's purpose
  Discriminating between statements of fact and statements of opinion
  Distinguishing between emotional and logical arguments
  Evaluating speaker's bias, prejudice, attitude

Metacognitive Level
  Monitoring of comprehension
  Recognizing when information is missing or incongruent
  Initiating repairs

Chapter 2, a person's motivation, interests, attitudes, and mood influence real-life comprehension. These issues need to be considered in assessing performance.

In addition, as discussed above, characteristics of the stimulus being presented must be considered. Table 3-9 lists the various stimulus characteristics that directly affect the difficulty of a listening task (Rost, 1990). These variables include the rate at which the information is presented, the length of the presentation, the number of informational units, the density of new information (degree of familiarity with content), and abstractness and redundancy of the content. The type of discourse is important because a descriptive discourse (list of descriptors or static traits) is easier to comprehend than a narrative (dynamic events that unfold in time), which, in turn, is easier to comprehend than expository discourse (such as an encyclopedia selection) (Rost, 1990).

An additional consideration is the amount of structure provided. Individuals process discourse that has semantic consistency and is well organized better than a poorly organized discourse with internal inconsistencies or inconsistencies with world knowledge. The linguistic complexity

Table 3-9.   Factors affecting the difficulty of a listening task.

Rate of speech

Length of stimulus

Number of informational units

Density of new information

Abstractness of content

Amount of redundancy and repetition

Type of discourse (static description—dynamic narrative—abstract expository discourse)

Amount of support or structure provided

Level of linguistic difficulty (vocabulary and syntax)

Appeal of topic

Background noise or distraction

in terms of vocabulary and syntactic structures is another variable in comprehension. An important factor, particularly after brain injury, is the relevance of given information to the person. Selections with topics of high interest to an individual tend to be listened to more intently.

A final consideration is the presence of background noise or distractions. Difficulty in monitoring and filtering irrelevant stimulation has been reported after TBI (Lezak, 1978), resulting in apprehension and anxiety in social situations in which the individual is bombarded by multiple sounds and input. Kewman, Yanus, and Kirsch (1988) find that individuals with TBI have greater difficulty comprehending spoken information in the presence of distracting vocal stimuli than under quiet conditions—substantially more so than do individuals without brain injury.

Methods for Assessing Listening

Keeping these listening skills and performance factors in mind, the clinician can then select the appropriate materials and methods for assessing functional comprehension. The most naturalistic method is to *measure listening in everyday settings*, especially in conversations with more than one person, in groups, or in community settings, such as on the job. The use of a checklist such as the one in Appendix E directs observations of behaviors pertinent to listening skills. Because it is an internal process rather than a true product, comprehension in natural settings must sometimes be inferred through an individual's responses in interactions.

Another strategy for assessing listening is to use *audio- or videotaped stimuli* from everyday life, such as a newscast, commercial, sports report, weather report, or another excerpt from a TV program or conversation. It is important to keep the selection short (about 1 to 2 minutes) to prevent overload of the individual's memory. The clinician can develop yes/no questions to measure comprehension and retention of main ideas and supporting details. Questions requiring the recall of information and tapping additional listening skills from Table 3–8 can be devised, as well.

A third method is to present *spoken passages* of various levels of complexity and ask questions concerning the passages, again tapping aspects of the listening skills in Table 3–8. Background noise may be introduced to a listening task to determine the ability to focus and control attention when effort must be applied. In addition, the rate of presentation can be varied, to determine optimal speed for successful processing.

If the individual is returning to an academic environment, it is important to simulate the listening demands of a classroom, presenting a spoken lecture at an appropriate level of complexity. The ability to comprehend information and to take meaningful notes from lectures should be assessed.

Brookshire and Nicholas (1993) developed a test to assess the comprehension of stated and implied main ideas and details from 10 stories. A yes/no question format is used to assess listening and reading comprehension and retention of these stories.

A fourth method to evaluate functional listening is to measure comprehension and retention of *spoken messages*. These can be assessed through the use of real or simulated phone calls. The individual's ability to comprehend and write down the important wh- information (*who, what, when, where,* and *why*) and phone numbers should be determined.

A fifth method for assessing functional comprehension is by asking the individual to execute *spoken directions* of various types. Comprehension of instructions is a complex task, requiring understanding of spatial (e.g., *between, right, down*) and deictic (e.g., *bring, take*) terms and complex logical-grammatical relationships (*before-after, if-then*) and retention of multiple steps in a particular sequence. Different types of directions have different response demands: following directions on a map, following directions to make a particular graphic design or written response, following directions for completing a route (within a building or in a city), or following instructions to complete a series of actions to produce a product (e.g., preparing food, playing a game, constructing a craft item).

In both of the latter two methods, assessment can be made of the metacognitive aspects of listening—factors extremely relevant to functional abilities. An individual's ability to handle the normal rate of speaking and to spontaneously use strategies when difficulty is experienced should be examined. Messages that are incomplete, ambiguous, or incomprehensible can be presented to determine if the individual is monitoring comprehension and can initiate a repair (Holland, 1980).

Assessing Speaking/Conversational Skills

Discourse abilities after brain injury have been found to vary with the setting or task (Brooks et al., 1987; Hartley & Jensen, 1991; Liles et al., 1989; Mentis & Prutting, 1987). Because of the variability both within and among individuals with brain injuries, no single method of assessment is sufficient to obtain a true picture of functional abilities. Techniques from pragmatics, behavioral assessment of social skills, ethnography, and discourse analysis should be combined to obtain a complete picture.

Observation of Natural Performance

A key method for assessing conversational or functional speaking abilities is *naturalistic observation.* Observation in multiple settings with multiple partners is generally the best strategy. The needs assessment or interviews should have suggested the environments and persons of relevance to a particular individual. Of primary consideration are those behaviors or situations that are felt to be most penalizing socially for the individual. When a particular environment has been identified as a difficult situation for the individual, the clinician should make direct observations in that setting. Checklists of various dimensions of social communication, such as those presented later in this section, can be used to facilitate data collection.

Observation in natural settings as an assessment method has face and ecological validity, but includes the disadvantage of requiring clinician time and transportation. When it is not feasible for the clinician to observe in multiple or real-life settings, input must be sought from persons who are very familiar with the individual's communication in social situations. The importance of obtaining input through an interview of a family member, friend, teacher, or co-worker was covered in a previous section. Completion of checklists or inventories by these individuals is another possible method for obtaining information. Goldstein et al. (1980) and Wiig (1982a) provide forms for having collateral sources indicate the frequency of use of various social skills, such as asking a favor or initiating a conversation. These provide quick and easy means to identify strengths and needs. The disadvantage is that the reliability and validity of the information depends on how familiar a collateral source is with the individual. Parents may not have had opportunities to observe an individual in more demanding situations, such as on the job or at school.

Observation of Unstructured Conversation With Clinician

A second major method of evaluating everyday speaking is through systematic *observations of unstructured conversation in a clinical setting.* The Pragmatic Protocol (Prutting & Kirchner, 1983, 1987; Milton et al., 1984) was developed as a screening tool for assessing conversation. Thirty communicative behaviors are judged as either appropriate (i.e., the behavior facilitated the interaction or was neutral) or inappropriate (i.e., the behavior detracted from the interchange and penalized the speaker). Definitions and appropriate versus inappropriate examples of each behavior are listed in Prutting and Kirchner (1987). To assess the individual, he or she is videotaped in an unstructured conversation with a familiar person for about 15 minutes. The Pragmatic Protocol, given in Appendix F, offers a quick, versatile system for guiding the clinician in videotape review to identify behaviors that penalize an individual or that facilitate interaction. This protocol could also be used in recording observations in real-life settings.

Use of Role Plays

The third major method for evaluating everyday social communication is through use of *analogue situations, or role-playing*. Simulation of life situations permits the manipulation of the environment to provide opportunities to observe behaviors of interest to the clinician. This is the approach used by Holland (1980) to assess the functional communication abilities of adults with aphasia and by Wiig (1982b) to assess the social skills of adolescents.

Simulation of social encounters or difficult social situations has been used frequently in behavioral assessment and interpersonal communication research. These situations generally have an individual initiating conversation and getting to know another person (often a member of the opposite sex) who is instructed to be minimally responsive (Farrell et al., 1985; Wallander, Conger, & Conger, 1985). The various "pretend" social settings include a restaurant on a blind date, a waiting room, and a snack bar (Conger et al., 1989). Wiig (1982a) provides suggestions for real-life situations that can be used to elicit different communicative intents or social skills through role play.

Role-playing is a way to evaluate the status of an individual's scripts, or knowledge of routine life activities, such as ordering pizza, making a doctor's appointment, or making airline reservations. Work-related communication tasks can be assessed through role play, as well (Groher, 1990).

Rating Scales of Conversational Abilities

Ehrlich and his colleagues have produced two rating scales that are adaptations of the Pragmatic Protocol. Pragmatic behaviors felt to be most relevant to persons with brain injuries were selected. The Communication Performance Scale (Ehrlich & Sipes, 1985), shown in Figure 3–2, was developed to rate 13 aspects of conversational abilities on a 1 to 5 scale. The reliability of this scale has not been addressed, but it provides an easy tool for the clinician to estimate the severity as well as the presence of an area of need.

Name: _____   Date: _____

1. *Intelligibility*
   difficult to understand   1   2   3   4   5   always understandable
   requires repetition

2. *Prosody/rate*
   choppy rhythm, uneven;   1   2   3   4   5   appropriate stress patterns
   too fast or slow

3. *Body Posture*
   away from others   1   2   3   4   5   body oriented towards others;
   limited gestures   appropriate gestures

4. *Facial Expression*
   limited affect and eye gaze   1   2   3   4   5   shows emotions and appropriate eye gaze

5. *Lexical Selection*
   limited word selection   1   2   3   4   5   good variety of words
   ambiguous words   clear referents

6. *Syntax*
   ungrammatical;   1   2   3   4   5   uses mature sentence patterns, phrases,
   uses only short phrases   clauses and conjunctions

7. *Cohesiveness*
   random, diffuse, and   1   2   3   4   5   planned, sequential expression of ideas;
   disjointed verbal style   concise

8. *Variety of Language Uses*
   limited use of language;   1   2   3   4   5   uses language to express feelings,
   stereotypical language   share information, social interaction

9. *Topic*
   abrupt shift of topic;   1   2   3   4   5   can appropriately introduce, maintain,
   perseveration   and change topic

10. *Initiation of Conversation*
    limited initiation of talk;   1   2   3   4   5   freely initiates and responds to
    restricted response to conversation   conversational leads

11. *Repair*
    inflexible, unable to change message   1   2   3   4   5   able to revise message to facilitate
    when communication failure occurs   listener comprehension; flexible

12. *Interruption*
    frequently interrupts others   1   2   3   4   5   appropriate interruption;
                                                            good conversation flow

13. *Listening*
    limited listening;   1   2   3   4   5   attends well;
    listener shows restricted reaction   listener provides verbal and non-verbal
    to the speaker   feedback to speaker

Figure 3-2.   Scale for rating conversational ability. (*Note*: From "Group Treatment of Communication Skills for Head Trauma Patients" by J. Ehrlich and A. Sipes, 1985, *Cognitive Rehabilitation*, 3, p. 37. Copyright 1985 by NeuroScience Publishers. Reprinted by permission.)

Ehrlich and Barry (1989) present a 9-point rating scale for assessing the quality of spontaneous conversation after brain injury. As shown in Table 3-10, five anchor points along the continuum are defined for six communicative behaviors: intelligibility, eye gaze, sentence formation, coherence

Table 3-10.   Conversational Rating Scale.

Intellgibility: Scale 1–9

1. Speech is severely distorted and consistently requires repetition
3. Speech is moderately distorted; can be understood approximately 30-40% of the time
5. Speech is mildly distorted; requires repetition approximately 10% of the time
7. Speech is minimally impaired, but is generally intelligible
9. No discernible speech impairment; always understood

Eye Gaze: Scale 1–9

1. Consistently no appropriate eye gaze with another person
3. Severely restricted eye gaze
5. Appropriate eye gaze 50% of the time
7. Appropriate eye gaze 75% of the time
9. Consistent use of appropriate eye gaze

Sentence Formation: Scale 1–9

1. Consistently uses ungrammatical sentences; only short phrases and "telegraphic"
3. Omits grammatical function words often; average sentence length is reduced most of the time
5. Uses mainly simple sentences; infrequent embedding and clauses
7. Uses varied sentence patterns 75% of the time
9. Mature and varied sentence patterns consistently used

Coherence of Narrative: Scale 1–9

1. Consistently random and diffuse expression; incomplete thoughts
3. Disjointed verbal style; limited connection between ideas
5. Thoughts are expressed with a moderate amount of irrelevant and extraneous remarks, and are considered incomplete 50% of the time
7. Ideas are expressed in some order approximately 75% of the time; notice occasional incomplete thoughts
9. Shows a well-executed expression of ideas most of the time; a well-formed narrative

Topic: Scale 1–9

1. Rapid and abrupt shifting from topic to topic within a short time
3. Able to maintain topic for at least 30 seconds
5. Can maintain topic for several minutes, but demonstrates difficulty in changing to a new topic
7. Can appropriately maintain the topic most of the time; infrequently (25% of the time) shows slowness and difficulty in change of topic
9. Demonstrates no problem in maintenance and change of topic

Initiation of Communication: Scale 1–9
   1. Infrequently initiates talk; only responds to others' questions
   3. Seldom initiates talk (about 25% of the time)
   5. Limited initiation of talk (about 50% of the time)
   7. Minimal problem in initiating conversational talk
   9. Freely initiates talk; good balance of communication most of the time

Note: From "Rating Communication Behaviours in the Head-Injured Adult" by J. Ehrlich and P. Barry, 1989, *Brain Injury, 3,* pp. 197–198. Copyright 1989 by Taylor and Francis. Reprinted by permission.

of narrative, topic, and initiation of communication. Adequate intra- and interrater reliability for this scale has been demonstrated.

The Behaviorally Referenced Rating System of Intermediate Social Skills (BRISS) was developed by Wallenger et al. (1985) to provide behavioral anchors for rating 11 behaviors on a 7-point scale. The behaviors include head movements, facial expression, involvement of the eyes, involvement of the arms and hands, overall body and leg movement, language expression, speech delivery (paralinguistics), conversation structure (turn taking), conversation content (topic), conversational style (humor, self-disclosure, and politeness), and partner-directed behavior (facilitation of partner's involvement). The BRISS was used by Marsh and Knight (1991) to measure social competence after brain injury.

Another useful rating scale was developed by Spitzberg and his colleagues (Spitzberg, 1983; Spitzberg & Hurt, 1987; Spitzberg & Huwe, 1991) for assessing the communicative competence of students enrolled in speech classes. As shown in Appendix G, the Conversational Skills Rating Scale (CSRS) consists of 25 items that are mainly at the molecular level of analysis and 5 items for rating global performance. Each item is rated on a 5-point scale, with a score of 1 indicating inadequate performance (resulting in a negative impression), 3 indicating adequate or sufficient performance, and 5 indicating an excellent performance that resulted in a positive impression of smooth, controlled skill in that area.

The CSRS was designed for ratings to be obtained from an individual, a communication partner, or an observer in either real-life or simulated situations. A factor analysis (Spitzberg, Brookshire, & Brunner, 1990) indicated that the 25 skills of the CSRS fall into five skill clusters, classified as interaction management (e.g., topic initiation, topic maintenance, interruptions), altercentrism (e.g., seeking clarification, reference to partner), expressiveness (e.g., vocal variety, gestures, expression of personal opinion), composure (e.g., vocal tension, unmotivated movements) and vocalics (e.g., articulation, rate, and fluency).

Burns, Halper, and Mogil (1985) designed a pragmatic rating scale to be used with patients with right hemisphere damage that has relevance to brain injury rehabilitation. Twelve behaviors are rated on a 1-to-5 scale from the categories of nonverbal communication, conversational skills (initiation, turn taking, and verbosity), use of linguistic context (topic maintenance, presupposition, and reference), and organization.

The use of rating scales and checklists in either natural or simulated conversation provides an efficient method of gathering and summarizing information about social behaviors at the intermediate-to-global level. Such lists can be used in a variety of natural and simulated life situations. Simplified versions can be used with clients for self-rating and self-monitoring of social interactions. To more discretely determine patterns of disruption, these techniques, however, often must be supplemented with more detailed analyses of cognitive-communicative performance, particularly in semantic aspects of communication.

Topic Analysis

Methods for analyzing topic initiation and maintenance have been recently developed to provide a more in-depth evaluation of conversation (Bedrosian, 1985, 1993; Mentis & Prutting, 1991). Mentis and Prutting (1991) define topic as "a clause or noun phrase that identified the question of immediate concern and that provided a global description of the content of a sequence of utterances" (p. 585). By focusing on topic, the sequential organization of conversation, the coordination of meaning, the initiation of communication, and coherence of the discourse can be examined. A worksheet for analyzing aspects of topic initiation, maintenance, and disruptions, adapted from Bedrosian (1985, 1993) and Mentis and Prutting (1991), is in Appendix H.

Both conversations and monologues (e.g., narratives, descriptive discourse) can be used as the basis of a topic analysis. Mentis and Prutting (1991) used six conversational samples and four monologues for one control and one individual with brain injury. Bedrosian (1985) videotaped and transcribed 10-minute conversations of individuals with severe language disorders with two different partners. Bedrosian (1993) recommends observing topic skills in 10-minute interactions with each of the following participants: a peer, an adult significant other, and a peer plus speech-language pathologist.

A topic analysis of each conversation is conducted by tallying each utterance under one of three categories—topic initiation, topic maintenance, and topic disruption (Bedrosian, 1993) on a form such as the one in Appendix H. Bedrosian (1993) recommends examining each topic initiation in 4 areas—subject matter, participant orientation, communicative intent, and outcome (successful or unsuccessful attempt to introduce a topic). Appendix H lists only the first three because they are the most relevant for individuals with TBI.

The category of subject matter is employed to determine if an individual initiates topics that are appropriate with a given partner. Each topic initiation is tallied as to whether the subject matter concerns a totally new, appropriate topic, represents a slight topic drift that continues to be relevant, or represents the introduction of an old topic. Next, the utterance is examined as to the participation orientation, that is, whether the topic focuses on the speaker, on another person, or on the speaker and another person (Bedrosian, 1993). This step is relevant to brain injury rehabilitation, because many times, an individual with TBI talks about himself or herself and does not ask about the partner (Marsh & Knight, 1992). Finally, each topic initiation is coded by the communicative intent, whether it provides information and does not require a response or whether it obliges the partner to respond. Topic is more easily established when a speaker initiates it with an utterance that requests information or action, instead of a declarative statement.

Topic maintenance is the second area for analysis of topic. Responses to topic initiations are examined and tallied on a form such as Appendix H. Continuation of a conversation generally entails the development of a topic through the use of requests for more information or the addition of new and relevant information. Minimal responses, such as in answering a question briefly, showing agreement/disagreement, and giving nonverbal or verbal acknowledgments, do not encourage interaction.

The third area of topic analysis examines disruptions in the flow of information. Characteristic error patterns, such as abrupt topic changes, ambiguous utterances, and irrelevant statements, can be detected by this step.

Error Analysis

Another approach for conducting a more in-depth analysis of conversational discourse is that used by Damico (1991) and Adams and Bishop (1989) (Bishop & Adams, 1989). Based on samples taken from conversations of a large group of children with language disabilities, they each created a system for categorizing errors that were noted, instances where the behavior was felt to be inappropriate or to adversely mark a child's communicative effectiveness.

As shown in Table 3–11, Damico (1991) organized his error analysis around Grice's (1975) maxims (discussed in Chapter 2). A conversational sample is first tape recorded and transcribed. Then, each utterance is tallied as either having a discourse problem or not on the Clinical Discourse Analysis form shown in Table 3–11. Each discourse error is identified on the form to provide a description of the individual's discourse ability. The percentage of utterances with problems provides an overall view of discourse performance.

Table 3–11. Clinical Discourse Analysis worksheet.

Quantity	_____
Insufficient information	_____
Nonspecific vocabulary	_____
Informational redundancy	_____
Need for repetition	_____
Quality	_____
Message inaccuracy	_____
Relation	_____
Poor topic maintenance	_____
Inappropriate response	_____
Failure to ask relevant questions	_____
Situational inappropriateness	_____
Inappropriate speech style	_____
Manner	_____
Linguistic nonfluency	_____
Revision	_____
Delay before responding	_____
Failure to structure discourse	_____
Turn-taking difficulty	_____
Gaze inefficiency	_____
Inappropriate intonational contour	_____
Total Utterances	_____
Total Discourse Problem Behaviors	_____
Total Utterances With These Behaviors	_____
Percentage of Utterances with Problem Behaviors	_____

Note: From "Clinical Discourse Analysis: A Functional Approach to Language Assessment" (p. 131) by J. S. Damico, 1991. In C. Simon (Ed.), *Communication Skills and Classroom Success: Assessment and Therapy Methodologies for Language and Learning Disabled Students.* Eau Claire, WI: Thinking Publications. Copyright 1991 by Thinking Publications. Reprinted by permission.

The inappropriate behaviors noted by Bishop and Adams (1989) are listed in Table 3–12. Each behavior was specifically defined and adequate interrater reliability was determined for most categories. Their taxonomy includes errors in comprehension as well as production.

An error analysis approach has relevance to functional goal setting for treatment, because behaviors that interfere with interpersonal communication are identified. This process, however, offers more of a descriptive rather than quantitative approach to assessment.

Analysis of Monologic Discourse

A fourth method of evaluating everyday communication is through *elicitation and analysis of monologic discourse* (as opposed to conversation) in the

Table 3-12. Categories of inappropriate responses in discourse of language-impaired children.

Expressive problems in semantics/syntax

Failure to comprehend literal meaning

Failure to respond to partner

Failure to use context in comprehension

Too little information provided
     Inappropriate presupposition
     Unestablished referent
     Logical step omitted

Too much information provided
     Unnecessary assertion/denial
     Excessive elaboration
     Unnecessary reiteration
     Ellipsis/reference not used when appropriate

Unusual or socially inappropriate content
     Topic drift (connected but irrelevant)
     Unmarked topic change
     Stereotypic phrases
     Inappropriate questioning (answer known or intent unclear)
     Socially inappropriate response (too personal)
     Inappropriate answer due to lack of knowledge/experience

Note: From "Conversational Characteristics of Children with Semantic-Pragmatic Disorder. II: What Features Lead to a Judgement of Inappropriacy?" by D. V. M. Bishop and C. Adams, 1989, *British Journal of Disorders of Communication,* 24, p. 246. Copyright 1989 by Whurr Publishers, Limited. Reprinted by permission.

clinical setting. In this approach, the clinician provides a stimulus, such as a picture or a goal, to obtain a sample of connected speech. Quantitative measures then are taken to more carefully determine an individual's ability to convey information in an organized and coherent manner.

This approach is more molecular in nature and, therefore, is more time consuming. It also requires greater knowledge of special techniques by the clinician. It has the advantage, however, of providing more objective data than some of the previous methods, with the clinician more able to precisely measure aspects of quantity, clarity, organization, and connectedness of discourse. These measures have been found to be very sensitive for detecting communication disorders after brain injury and for providing clinically relevant information (Cannito, Hayashi, & Ulatowska, 1988; Coehlo et al., 1991a, 1991b, 1991c; Hartley & Jensen, 1991, 1992; Liles et al., 1989; Mentis & Prutting, 1987). This method also permits greater clinician control of the type of discourse and complexity of ideas to be conveyed. Many individuals with brain injuries perform within normal limits in casual conversation, but experience difficulty when the topic is controlled by another person or when a particular type of discourse is required (Marsh & Knight, 1991; Mentis & Prutting, 1987).

Types of Monologic Discourse. Three types of monologic discourse have typically been elicited for analysis: descriptive, narrative, and procedural discourse. The "Cookie Theft Picture" from the *Boston Diagnostic Aphasia Examination* (Goodglass & Kaplan, 1983) is frequently used to elicit a picture description. Norms for determining the number of content units (vocabulary items) were provided in Yorkston and Beukelman (1980). Qualitative judgments can be made of an individual's awareness of causal relations, interpretation and integration of complex visual information, and word retrieval in connected speech. This task, however, is relatively easy for individuals with brain injuries. Ehrlich (1988) found that individuals with TBI generated the same number of content units as did normal speakers on this task. They were, however, less efficient, taking longer to produce the same amount of information.

A narrative, or story, is a discourse that consists of characters and episodes in which events and actions unfold in time. Much of our relationship-building conversations consists of narratives. People use narratives to recount their daily experiences or tell of something they heard on the TV or read in the newspaper. They discuss their future plans or tell of past events. The use of narratives involves many of the skills necessary in interpersonal communication: attribution of motivation, identification of feelings, understanding of cause-and-effect relationships, and knowledge of personal relationships.

Narratives can be elicited through the use of a series of pictures, such as a comic strip, or a complex picture, such as a Norman Rockwell painting. Other methods include having an individual retell a story heard from an audiotape, read, or seen on a videotape. Retelling a story is generally easier for a person with brain injury than generating a story from a visual stimulus (Hartley & Jensen, 1991; Liles et al., 1989).

The third type of discourse most often elicited, procedural discourse, consists of a series of steps organized in a temporal and hierarchical manner to tell someone how to do something. This can be elicited by asking the individual to tell how to perform an everyday activity (e.g., make a sandwich, change a flat tire, or buy groceries), how to get to a certain location, or how to perform some work-related task relevant to that individual. This task can reveal the ability of the individual to sequence and plan an activity.

Other types of monologic discourse include expository discourse (e.g., textbooks, encyclopedia articles) and persuasive discourse (stating an opinion and giving supporting information).

When using this approach, efforts should be made to ensure that tasks are as similar to real-life situations as possible (Hartley, 1990). That is, the task should be presented in a manner that discourages the individual from assuming that the examiner has previous knowledge of the stimulus. Videotapes or audiotapes should be presented without the clinician present. Visual material should be placed out of the direct view of the examiner, perhaps even with a barrier between the examiner and the picture.

Analysis of Monologic Discourse. Typically, the elicited spoken discourse is audiotaped and then transcribed to permit the tallying of various measures and to provide a permanent record. Written discourses can be analyzed in the same manner as spoken discourse. Measures that have been used include both sentential and discourse level analyses. As shown in Table 3–13, sentential measures include the average length of utterance, incomplete utterances, utterances with syntactic errors, or type of syntactic constructions used. Although individuals with TBI demonstrate relatively preserved syntactic abilities, they have been shown to make more grammatical errors at times or to use simpler sentence constructions than is typical of noninjured speakers (Hartley, 1986; Mentis & Prutting, 1987).

The discourse level measures that have been used, as shown in Table 3–13, include measures of productivity or fluency, semantic content, and cohesion. Productivity measures indicate the overall quantity of discourse produced and the ease with which an individual produces discourse. "Talkativeness" is quantified by measuring the speaking time, number of words produced, and number of utterances produced. The rate of speaking, measured in either words per minute or syllables per second, provides an indication of processing, or psychomotor speed, and/or problems in word retrieval. Mazes, or dysfluencies, are revisions, part- or whole-word repetitions, and filled pauses that reflect difficulty in putting thoughts into spoken words (Loban, 1976). After brain injury, the degree of maze behavior may indicate word retrieval, attention, or verbal planning problems (Hartley & Jensen, 1991; Penn & Cleary, 1988).

Because word retrieval is a common problem following brain injury, it is particularly important to determine how this affects functional communication or discourse abilities. Word-retrieval problems can affect all levels of discourse production. Marshall (1976) observes that adults with aphasia demonstrate five strategies to compensate for word-retrieval problems in connected speech: delay, semantic association, phonemic association, description, and generalization. Some individuals with severe word-retrieval problems following brain injury produce confabulatory responses, for example calling a canoe a "canoota" (Prigatano, Roueche, & Fordyce, 1986).

German (1987) looked at word finding in the discourse of children and developed categories of behaviors she believed to reflect word-finding problems. These included delays of 6 seconds or more, unnecessary repetitions of part or whole words, reformulations or grammatical revi-

Table 3–13. Quantitative measures of discourse production.

Sentential Measures
   Average length of utterances
   Number of incomplete utterances
   Number of utterances with incorrect syntax
   Type of syntactic construction
      Single clause
      Compound subject and/or predicate
      Complex

Measures of Productivity/Fluency
   Total speaking time
   Number of meaningful words
   Number of utterances
   Speaking rate
   Percentage of dysfluent productions

Measures of Semantic Content
   Organization of content
      Elements of discourse superstructure
   Quantity of content
      Number of content words (as in *The Boston Diagnostic Aphasia Examination*
         "Cookie Theft Picture")
      Number of propositions or main themes
   Problems in semantic content
      Number of inaccurate propositions
      Instances of problems in clarity of reference
      Errors in use of pronouns
      Indefinite words (*thing, stuff, something*)
      Naming errors
   Inappropriate content
      Irrelevant statements
      Personal experience/evaluation
      Excessive detail
      Redundant statements

Measures of Cohesion (Halliday & Hasan, 1976)
   Cohesive ties per utterance

Note: From "Assessment of Functional Communication" (p. 153) by L. Hartley. In D. Tupper and K. Cicerone (Eds.), *The Neuropsychology of Everyday Life, Vol. 1: Assessment and Basic Competencies,* 1990, Boston: Kluwer Academic Publishers. Copyright 1990 by Kluwer Academic. Adapted by permission.

sions of a phrase or changes in word selection, starter phrases used to initiate utterances (i.e., *and so*), incomplete phrases, fillers such as *um* or *er*, empty words or phrases (*thing, stuff, whatchama call it*), and grammatical errors. Paraphasias which substitute for a targeted word were also included.

The semantic content of a discourse can be analyzed in terms of its organization, quantity of information, and quality of information provided. Discourse "grammar" is the superstructure of the discourse consisting of essential and optional components. Narrative grammar was used by Labov (1972) and has been studied extensively by Ulatowska and associates. The elements of a narrative, described in Cannito et al. (1988), are:

1. Abstract (optional)—summarizes the whole story.
2. Setting—participants, time, and place.
3. Complicating action—events that happened to change the setting.
4. Result or resolution of events.
5. Evaluation—the point of the narrative.
6. Coda—signals the end.

The superstructure of a procedural discourse consists of an optional statement of purpose and a setting, followed by an ordered set of essential steps, with any nonessential steps (steps that clarify or provide details), and finally an optional coda or goal statement (Cannito et al., 1988; Graesser, 1978; Ulatowska, Freedman-Stern, Weiss, Macaluso-Haynes, & North, 1983; Ulatowska, North, & Macaluso-Haynes, 1981).

The quantity of content or information has been measured by examining the number of vocabulary terms used (Yorkston & Beukelman, 1980) or the number of themes or propositions used (Berko-Gleason et al., 1980; Hartley & Jensen, 1991). This measure quantifies the informativeness of the speaker's discourse.

As shown in Table 3–13, another way of analyzing the semantic content is to tally any problems. For persons with brain injuries, these errors usually include the use of false information, irrelevant statements, redundant information, excessive details, vague statements, or statements of personal experiences tangentially related to the discourse. One major problem frequently found after neurological damage is the lack of clarity of reference. Failures in achieving adequate reference to events or persons may be caused by word-finding difficulty (see German, 1987) or difficulties in perspective taking. The speaker may use pronouns without first providing the referent.

The last broad category of discourse measures is cohesive ties. The taxonomy of cohesion most often used is that of Halliday and Hasan (1976). These include reference, conjunction, ellipsis, substitution, and lexical cohesion. Table 3–14 provides definitions and examples of each of these types of cohesion.

For more complete information concerning analysis techniques, definitions, and examples, the reader is referred to Cannito et al. (1988); Coelho et al. (1991a, 1991b, 1991c); Hartley and Jensen (1991); Joanette and Brownell (1990); Liles et al. (1989); and Mentis and Prutting (1987).

Table 3–14.   Categories of cohesion derived from Halliday and Hasan (1976) with contrived examples.

Reference: Instances in which a word cannot be interpreted without reference to information in another clause.

Examples:	
Personal	Bob went to the store, but *it* was closed.
Demonstrative	A flower pot fell on his head and *that* made him angry.
	A car went speeding past us. We couldn't tell who was in *the* car.
Comparative	Roger gave the beggar all his money, but the beggar was not quite *so nice.*

Substitution: The replacement of a nominal, verbal, or clausal unit by another item having the same structural function as that of the item replaced.

Examples:	Jim said he would leave and he *did.*
	It's going to rain. At least the radio said *so.*

Ellipsis: An instance in which the clausal structure contains a slot to be filled by reference to preceding text.

Example:	Joe was the first person to arrive.
	I was the second.
	I can't come, but Lindsey will.

Conjunction: A word that specifies the way in which the utterance following it is related to what has gone before.

Examples:	
Additive	A man was walking *and* he found a wallet.
Adversative	The man said he would come, *but* he never did.
Causal	The girl was curious, *so* she opened the box.
Temporal	Jan finished the letter, *then* she went to the mailbox.

Lexical: The repetition of various vocabulary items to refer to a person, event, object, or fact.

Examples:	
Synonym	My friend called yesterday. What a great *pal!*
Subordinate	We bought a new vehicle. It's a *minivan.*
General	I read his report. The whole *thing* is inaccurate.

Assessment of Everyday Activities

Depending on the work setting and role of the speech-language pathologist on the rehabilitation team, evaluation of daily living and community activities may be an SLP responsibility, as well. The clinician can construct an assessment of an individual's ability to perform real-life activities, such as grocery shopping, eating in a fast food restaurant, or following a recipe, through observation of either real-life or simulated situations that are relevant to an individual's own needs, as determined by the needs assessment.

Because procedures and materials are not standardized, when making these types of naturalistic observations, the clinician must be conscious of various factors that affect an individual's performance (Milton & Wertz, 1986; Sohlberg & Mateer, 1989a). These factors can be divided into stimulus, response, and environmental characteristics. Through manipulation of these characteristics, the clinician can define an individual's present level of performance and pinpoint the factors that affect his or her performance of a particular task.

When constructing an assessment of a functional activity, the clinician must first decide the particular task to be assessed, the criteria against which performance will be judged, and the potential factors affecting performance (Sohlberg & Mateer, 1989a). A task analysis of an activity may be the first step to determine the steps expected in typical performance for that particular task. Falvey (1989) provides a task analysis for evaluating performance at a fast food restaurant. Sohlberg and Mateer (1989b) present an observational protocol for use in making a naturalistic assessment of meal preparation.

Some of the major task or stimulus parameters to be considered, synthesized from Haarbauer-Krupa, Moser, Smith, Sullivan, and Szekeres (1985); Milton and Wertz (1986); Sohlberg and Mateer (1989a); and Szekeres et al. (1987) are listed in Table 3–15. Each of these parameters can affect the difficulty of a task and must be carefully considered when constructing an assessment task.

The environmental characteristics that influence performance, taken again from the above references, are listed in Table 3–16. One primary consideration is the amount of clinician assistance in terms of cueing or prompting that must be provided for the individual to complete the task successfully. An adaptation of Falvey's (1989) hierarchy of cueing or prompting is shown in Table 3–17. The clinician should provide the least intrusive form of prompting that is necessary. Another consideration is to the amount of external structuring that is required. Performance may be optimal when certain restrictions are placed on the environment, as in a quiet environment, or when certain adaptations, such as checklists or use of a tape recorder, are made.

The final consideration deals with the response parameters for judging performance in functional activities. Table 3–18 lists possible ways of measuring performance variables. Other considerations are the cognitive aspects of performance—safety, problem solving, planning, sequencing, self-monitoring, and organization. Some aspects of performance can be assessed with a task analysis checklist. Though not a focus of this book, the effect of physical limitations, such as hemiparesis or dysarthria, on performance should be taken into account.

Summary

This chapter has described a number of methods for acquiring information about an individual's cognitive-communicative abilities after brain injury.

Table 3-15.   Task parameters to be manipulated in functional activities.

Parameter	Manipulation
Rate of presentation	Slow to fast
Length of stimulus	Short to long
Familiarity of stimulus	Familiar versus unfamiliar
Modality of presentation	Auditory versus visual
	Unimodal versus crossmodal
Content	Verbal versus nonverbal
	Nonmeaningful versus meaningful
Familiarity of stimuli	Familiar versus unfamiliar
Level of abstraction	Concrete versus abstract
Linguistic features	Simple versus complex syntax
	Low versus high level vocabulary
Units	Single versus multiple steps
Procedural complexity	Simple, structured versus complex,
(planning, organization, problem solving,	integrative, unstructured
decision-making involvement)	
Variability of stimuli	Consistent versus inconsistent form
	Consistent versus inconsistent occurrence
Visual complexity	Simple versus complex

Note: Based on material from Haarbauer-Krupa, Moser, Smith, Sullivan, and Szezeres, (1985); Milton and Wertz (1986), Sohlberg and Mateer (1989a); and Szekeres, Ylvisaker, and Cohen (1987).

Table 3-16.   Environmental factors to be manipulated or considered in judging functional performance.

Parameter	Manipulations
Cueing	Specific versus nonspecific
	Number of cues provided
	Verbal versus gestural prompts
Scope/Adaptability	Special adaptations or devices
	Controlled circumstances
	Structured versus unstructured environment
	Individual versus group setting
Stressors	Time constraints
	Temperature
	Noise/distractions
	Interruptions

Note: Based on material from Haarbauer-Krupa, Moser, Smith, Sullivan, and Szezeres, (1985); Milton and Wertz (1986); Sohlberg and Mateer (1989a); and Szekeres, Ylvisaker, and Cohen (1987).

Table 3-17. Hierarchy of prompting.

Level of Prompt	Behavior
Natural	No cue necessary
Gestural	Clinician points
Indirect verbal	Clinician provides nonspecific verbal prompt (e.g., "What else?")
Direct verbal	Clinician provides specific verbal instruction
Model	Clinician models, then gives person turn
Physical	Clinician provides minimal, moderate, or full physical assistance to complete a task

Note: From *Community-Based Curriculum: Instructional Strategies for Students With Severe Handicaps* (2nd ed.) (p. 78) by M. A. Falvey, 1989, Baltimore: Paul H. Brookes Publishing Co. Copyright 1989 by Paul H. Brookes Publishing Co. (P.O. Box 10624, Baltimore, MD 21285-0624). Adapted by permission.

Table 3-18. Response parameters to be measured during functional activities.

Parameter	Examples of Measures or Categories
Consistency/Accuracy	Percentage of correct responses
	Number of errors
Efficiency/Frequency	Latency of response
	Rate (amount per unit of time)
Duration	Total time
Intensity	Below normal, normal, above normal
Response mode	Oral, written, gestural, manipulative
Initiative	Performed or not performed
	Number of occurrences
Appropriateness	Appropriate versus inappropriate

Note: Based on material from Haarbauer-Krupa, Moser, Smith, Sullivan, and Szekeres (1985); Milton and Wertz (1986); and Sohlberg and Mateer (1989a).

The emphasis is on developing a complete picture of an individual's cognitive-communicative competence within his or her own social and cultural environment. Evaluation procedures must be balanced across the different levels of outcome, including impairment, functional limitations, and disability. Input from multiple sources must be synthesized to create a rich picture that is sensitive to environmental influences and personal needs, values, and preferences.

It is not feasible for one clinician to conduct all of these procedures in an initial evaluation. Therefore, an examiner must start with as broad a brush stroke as possible and continue to obtain information through diagnostic therapy or through shared responsibilities with other team members. At a minimum, however, the clinician should:

1. Review the records of an individual.
2. Obtain the perspective of the individual on his or her abilities, areas of need, and goals.
3. Obtain input from the family or significant others regarding cognitive-communication functioning.
4. Conduct standardized testing of cognitive-communicative processes and semantic knowledge, making use of clinical observations as well as standardized procedures.
5. Use checklists or rating scales to evaluate cognitive-communication in unstructured real-life activities.
6. Evaluate discourse comprehension and production.

The most difficult part of an evaluation is the integration and synthesis of information to form a cohesive picture of an individual, the current level of function, and the path for the future. Determining a diagnosis in terms of a unitary label is not so important with this population as much as a description of an individual's strengths and needs. As stated at the beginning of this chapter, the evaluation should help answer the following questions:

1. **Does the individual have a cognitive-communication disorder?** Data from all sources are needed to determine this. Neither standardized test scores nor informal procedures, alone, are sufficient. Knowledge of the level of premorbid functioning of the individual is critical, as well as the person's own perceptions of any changes. A diagnosis in terms of a specific label with this population, however, is not as important as the next step.

2. **What are the strengths and needs of the individual?** Use of both standardized and informal tests will identify the relative strengths and needs of the individual. However, information from the environmental needs assessment and interviews provides the basis for weighing these results and determining relevant social factors. Starting with the initial reason for the referral, the clinician should look for consistencies among the data to identify the nature and scope of the cognitive-communication challenges.

3. **What are the underlying causes of the changes in cognitive-communication abilities?** This is determined initially by case history and standardized test data. Observational data should be used to corroborate hypotheses and to determine environmental influences, as well.

4. **What is the prognosis for benefit from additional treatment?** As previously discussed, many factors contribute to outcome after TBI (refer to Figure 3–1). The major determinant is generally felt to be the

severity of injury. One indication of the severity of injury is the initial Glasgow Coma Scale (GCS) score. Of course, individuals with no coma (GCS greater than 8) have a better prognosis than those with a GCS less than 9. Another indication is the length of coma, with coma duration less than 24 hours being a positive prognostic indicator and greater than 2 weeks being a negative indicator. The history of any complications such as anoxia, increased intracranial pressure, seizures, and intracranial mass lesions requiring surgery are all negative factors. In terms of cognitive findings, persisting aphasia, poor complex attention, severe motor dysfunction, and lack of awareness are negative factors for community reintegration. Demographic characteristics are also considerations. Younger age is associated with a greater likelihood for return to employment and independent living for adults with brain injury. The higher the level of premorbid education and occupational status, the more likely is a return to work. Psychosocial factors associated with better outcomes include the presence of family and social support systems and the absence of a history of substance abuse, psychiatric disturbance, emotional instability, and legal problems. Personality characteristics, such as determination and self-motivation, are important. And the importance of a sense of humor cannot be overlooked, as well.

5. What should the plan of treatment include? The translation of evaluation findings into a treatment plan is a complex task, in itself. This is covered in the next chapter.

Finally, assessment of functional cognitive-communicative abilities is a dynamic and systematic process that requires sensitivity to relevant contexts of functional activities and collaboration with the individual being evaluated, family members, and other service providers. Reference to a sound model of cognitive-communicative abilities anchors this complex and rich process that seeks to identify themes and to capture the uniqueness and possibilities of each individual. This process allows the development of a personally and socially relevant treatment plan for an individual.

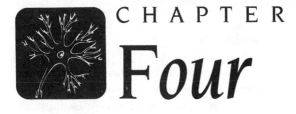

CHAPTER

Four

Functional Approaches to Cognitive-Communicative Treatment: Laying the Groundwork

The challenge of treatment planning and implementation is enormous after brain injury because the needs are so great and cross so many disciplines and situations. It is easy to get lost in the litany of needs and other assessment data and lose focus on the destination—community reintegration.

As Wood (1990) states so aptly, clinicians must always bear in mind that the purpose of rehabilitation is to reduce "the social handicap imposed by cognitive disability" (p. 4). Variations from individual to individual make treatment planning even more complex. There is no easy solution; no single manual exists that can explain the translation of assessment into treatment that will work in all instances. No one workbook can provide the treatment for all cases. Nevertheless, this chapter provides some guidelines and pointers for maintaining appropriate direction and focus.

General Principles of Treatment

Perhaps a good starting place is to identify some general principles of treatment for maintaining a functional approach. As listed in Table 4–1, the first principle is that cognitive-communicative intervention must be based on sound theory, with a firm conceptualization of dysfunction caused by brain injury, of normal information processing and learning, and of key dimensions of everyday communication. Chapter 2 provided a model of social communication to assist clinicians in framing treatment as well as evaluation.

The second principle is that rehabilitation at the postacute stage must be focused on functional adaptation, adjustment, and compensation rather than restoration of function (Milton & Wertz, 1986). Each individual must be assisted in obtaining as productive a life as possible through adjustment to impairments, compensation, and functional skill development.

The third principle is that the primary concern should be on meeting the functional needs of an individual and achieving the desired long-term outcomes. This means that the clinician must always bear in mind the time frames available, realistic discharge goals, and skills that are needed to obtain those goals (Whitman, 1991). Therefore, before a treatment plan can be fully developed, the team must be aware of discharge plans and options. Many of the key elements of discharge planning have been discussed as part of the case history and interviews of the individual and significant others sections. A method for solidifying this information into long-term goals, "Futures Planning," is discussed in the next section.

As stated in Chapter 1, a functional approach governs not only the philosophy and process of rehabilitation, but also the content. This means that materials and tasks should be selected based on an individual's functional needs and personal interests and preferences. For example, Sharon had persisting dyslexia and dysgraphia as a result of traumatic brain injury (TBI). Previous rehabilitation efforts had used reading workbooks in an attempt to reteach phonics. Sharon was bored and barely cooperative with this approach. During her evaluation, she had revealed that she wanted a better relationship with her 4-year-old daughter who had been living with the maternal grandmother in another town for the 2 years Sharon had been in various rehabilitation programs. Sharon became much more interested in working on her reading when children's books were selected as the vehicle for practice. The use of contextual cues from pictures as well as the surrounding text was emphasized. The treatment of her writing difficulties centered on her functional needs, including writing brief letters to her daughter. Several months into her postacute rehabilitation program, she went home for a holiday. She had tears in her eyes when

Table 4-1. Principles of treatment.

Intervention must be based on sound theory.

Treatment must be focused on functional adaptation, compensation, and adjustment, not restoration of function.

Treatment must be driven by functional needs and desired long-term outcomes.

Tasks should resemble real-life events.

Personal cognitive-communicative goals should be clearly defined, with interdisciplinary participation and consistent reinforcment throughout the day.

Family, peers, and others in the individual's social network should be brought into treatment process.

Self-evaluation and monitoring techniques should be included.

she returned, stating that for the first time since her injury, her daughter would sit in her lap. This happened because Sharon was able to read her stories and use this as a means of reestablishing their relationship.

The fourth principle in Table 4–1 is that therapy tasks should resemble real-life events as much as possible. Although it may be necessary to work on basic skills or processes, such as vocabulary or organization, thought should be given to the application and generalization of these skills within functional contexts. In this manner, treatment of cognitive processes and functional skills should be blended to facilitate application of compensatory strategies to actual life situations. In addition, whenever possible, treatment should be conducted in natural contexts.

A fifth principle is that each individual must have clearly defined personal cognitive-communicative goals that are consistently reinforced throughout the treatment day. The goals should be short and meaningful to the individual, as "Get to the point," "Speak up," or "Think first." Close interdisciplinary collaboration and client participation are important in setting these goals. This means that an individual is made aware of the needs in communication and that the desired behavior is objectively defined. It also means that the entire team, not just one discipline, is responsible for working on social communication, so that consistent reinforcement is achieved throughout an individual's day.

The sixth principle is related to the fifth in that all persons around the individual should be included in treatment planning and implementation. This means that family, significant others, friends, co-workers, and peers in the rehabilitation program should all be part of the "milieu," helping to integrate the person back into society. One of the purposes is to reduce the reliance on therapist feedback and place more emphasis on natural supports and relationships.

A final principle is that monitoring and self-evaluation techniques must be incorporated into all aspects of treatment. The individual must be trained to evaluate the performance of others and him- or herself to develop the ability to monitor performance in real-life situations. Implicit in this is an individual's understanding of the areas being targeted and acceptance of the need to work on those areas.

Long-Term Goal Setting

The first step in a functional approach to treatment planning is identification of the desired outcomes (Whitman, 1991). Information gained in the assessment process must be pulled together and the significant players must determine the target destination for an individual.

Input must come from a number of sources. The funding source representative must be involved to establish acceptable time frames for funding and desired outcomes from the payer's point of view. The team input from the interdisciplinary evaluation is important to determine realistic expectations for progress and what an individual can accomplish within the given program. The family's input is critical because of the important emotional, social, psychological, physical, problem-solving, and financial support they provide. Significant others, such as friends, also can be included in the process. The input of the individual is, of course, of supreme importance. This is essential to empowerment of the individual; the individual is assisted in the identification of options and in the determination of his or her desired outcomes for rehabilitation.

Futures Planning is a procedure developed by a nonprofit case management firm, Independent Case Management, Inc., of Little Rock, Arkansas, to assist families and persons with disabilities in determining long-range goals and organizing resources to achieve the preferred future. It is conducted through discussions with all persons listed above. A related process is that of Willer, Allen, Anthony, and Cowlan (1993) called "Circle of Support." Its purpose is to identify a natural support system to work together to help an individual with brain injury achieve his or her aspirations. The individual selects persons in his or her support system who will meet periodically and assist in identifying resources and possibilities for more complete community reintegration.

The first step in Futures Planning is to gather information, using a form such as the one in Appendix I from the author's center, concerning an individual's past, present, and future. The planning session begins with capturing a snapshot view of a person's past, of significant life events, and how a person has evolved to his or her current life situation. Then locations in the discharge or current community that are a part of an individual's life are listed as an indication of the degree of community participation, areas of interest, lifestyle, training needs, and possible resources and support networks. The next step is to identify the significant people in an individual's life. This helps in making an individual and team aware of persons available as resources, such as leads for job seeking, assistance in transportation to work or going on leisure outings, or friends to reinforce adaptive social behaviors. This identifies a circle of support for an individual.

By the time of postacute rehabilitation, many individuals with brain injury feel that they have been stripped of all decision-making authority and that others control every aspect of their lives. Some individuals may have acquired a learned helplessness, feeling incapable of making decisions. The futures planning helps them identify the current choices they have in daily activities, such as what to wear, what to buy, and what to eat, as well as in their rehabilitation program, such as treatment goals, leisure activities, and options for treatment. By examining what they like and dislike, individuals can better identify ways to achieve a rewarding future and staff can understand better what motivates an individual.

As shown in Appendix I, the next step in the futures planning is to use the input of all persons, especially the individual with brain injury, to determine the desired future in each life domain. The emphasis is on the positive and the future—but the identified goals still must be realistic. Although not included on the form, financial aspects should be considered, as well, to ensure adequate resources for the future.

The strengths of a person that will assist in achieving the desired goals are then identified, followed by any obstacles or hurdles that might stand in the way. An action plan is then formulated, with persons responsible and dates for completion established.

This process of long-term goal setting is important for active engagement of an individual from the very beginning in determining the outcome goals of rehabilitation and empowering the individual to make informed decisions about his or her future. Once all the players involved in the management of an individual have decided on the long-term goals, the treatment team amalgamates this information with the evaluation results to formulate a program plan that will assist the individual in achieving those outcome goals step-by-step.

Overview of Models of Intervention

Few studies exist on the relative efficacy of the different treatment approaches following brain injury. In general, clinicians combine treatment models, with the major intervention strategy varying according to the stage of recovery and the severity of injury. An overview of intervention models is presented here to promote understanding of the options for treatment and how treatment meshes with the three levels of injury outcome evaluation—impairment, functional limitation (or disability), and handicap as discussed in Chapter 3 (see Figure 3–1). A more in-depth discussion of the treatment models relevant to postacute rehabilitation is included in the next chapter.

Facilitation-Stimulation

As shown in Table 4–2, the first model of cognitive-communicative intervention is facilitation-stimulation. Facilitation-stimulation techniques are aimed at maximizing recovery by stimulating an individual at a level that permits optimal processing and performance. Treatment in this model consists of graded activities to increase alertness, understanding of the environment, and the variety of adaptive behaviors (Smith & Ylvisaker, 1985). This is the model of intervention that dominates early treatment after injury, but it is not considered a major treatment strategy for later stages of recovery (Haarbauer-Krupa, Henry, Szekeres, & Ylvisaker, 1985).

Component Process Retraining

Component process retraining is aimed at improving a person's specific impairments or the cognitive or language processes that are defective due to brain injury. Treament may consist of drills or exercises designed to improve an isolated cognitive-communicative function, such as selective attention or word finding, determined to be impaired through standardized testing. This model is based on the belief that deficit areas can be improved through training in those areas.

Environmental Manipulation

Environmental manipulation, or modification of an individual's social or physical environment, is the third treatment model listed in Table 4–2.

Table 4–2.   Models of cognitive-communicative intervention.

Facilitation-stimulation

Component process retraining

Environmental manipulation

Compensatory strategy training

Functional-integrative skill training

Stimulus-response conditioning

Modifications may serve to suppress undesirable behaviors, make existing behaviors adequate, or prompt the use of new adaptive responses (Gross & Schutz, 1986). This model acknowledges that behavior is the result of interaction between the individual and his or her environment. Through appropriate supports or changes in the environment, an individual may be able to perform satisfactorily despite impairments. No learning by the individual is required in this model. Concrete examples include setting up a quiet study area for the person that is free of distractions to overcome attentional deficits or the labeling of drawers or cabinets to overcome memory deficits. Another strategy is to train supervisors and co-workers in ways to interact with the individual to avoid behavior challenges.

Compensatory Strategy Training

The fourth model involves personal compensation for areas of weakness by making use of retained abilities. The purpose of this model is not to improve the areas of deficit, but to teach the individual to overcome them through employment of internal compensatory strategies or external aids. Examples include teaching individuals to write information down rather than rely on their memory and to ask for repetition of instructions when they do not understand.

Functional Skills Training

The fifth model is functional skills training or training of functional-integrative skills (Gross & Schultz, 1986; Szekeres, Ylvisaker, & Holland, 1985). In this model, functional skills rather than component processes are the focus of intervention. This model is based on the assumption that functional skills can be improved through learning and practice. Treatment is often conducted in functional settings. Activities in this model include training in making telephone calls, writing checks, or conversing with others.

Stimulus-Response Conditioning

The final model is the use of behavior modification principles to reinforce or discourage discrete behaviors to increase functioning in the person's environment (Gross & Schultz, 1986; Giles & Clark-Wilson, 1993; Jacobs, 1993). This approach is also a methodology through which functional skills, component processes, or compensatory strategies can be taught. Examples include use of social praise to reinforce adaptive behavior and withdrawal of attention or privileges to reduce maladaptive or undesirable behaviors.

Developing a Functional Treatment Plan

The development of a functional treatment plan depends on many factors, including the scope of the rehabilitation program and the disciplines involved. Goal formulation is particularly difficult when treatment is aimed at decreasing functional limitations or disability and enhancing community reintegration. Goals need to be objective and measurable, as well as functionally meaningful. Input from all the evaluation steps and from the Futures Planning are combined to establish treatment goals at three levels of function, the macro, middle, and micro (Ramsberger, 1994; Wilkerson, 1992). These levels correspond to Nagi's (1969) levels of disability, functional limitation, and impairment, respectively, as discussed in Chapter 3.

The first step in developing the treatment plan is to use the input from the Futures Planning and all the evaluation procedures to identify and agree on the targeted long-term outcomes for each life domain. For example, what is the realistic and expected living outcome for the individual? The outcome goal for an individual with severe cognitive and physical challenges may be to be able to live in a group home. The desired goal for another individual with moderate memory and mild language deficits may be to live at home with a spouse with minimal assistance and supervision. These outcome goals address the macro level of functioning and seek to decrease a person's disability.

The second step is to identify intermediate goals at the middle level of function. These come from the environmental needs assessment, from a task analysis of the everyday activities in a particular environment, through interview of the individual or family, or through other assessment procedures. These goals address the functional components that lead up to the desired outcome goal. Examples of these goals are shown in Table 4–3.

The next step in developing a functional treatment plan is to identify short-term (generally monthly) objectives at the micro level of function. These goals can be stated from a process perspective or from a functional skill perspective. Examples of short-term goals are presented in Table 4–3.

The goals in Appendix J were developed more from a process point of view or, borrowing from educational terminology, a statement of minimal competency. Descriptors must be added to define the stimulus, response, and environmental characteristics that form the basis for judging successful performance. These considerations were listed in Tables 3–15, 3–16, and 3–18. For example, a goal statement might be that an individual will state the main idea and one supporting detail from a concrete, four-sentence spoken expository paragraph in a quiet environment with 100% accuracy in four out of five trials.

Another approach to goal setting is to focus on the communication skills actually required in the functional activities found to be a part of the

Table 4-3.   Example of a functional program plan for an individual with moderate memory and mild language deficits.

Functional Life Domain: Independent Living

Outcome Goal: To live at home with her husband with only minimal assistance and intermittent supervision.

Intermediate Goals	Short-Term Objectives
1. She will be able to access emergency medical system.	**1a.** She will dial 911 correctly. **1b.** She will state the problem in role plays of emergency situations.
2. She will use her memory notebook to retrieve personal and orientation information.	**2a.** She will locate names of family members in her notebook when unable to name pictures spontaneously. **2b.** She will use her calendar to determine day of week, date, and scheduled events.
3. She will be able to use the telephone independently to make routine calls.	**3a.** She will be able to locate frequently used phone numbers in her address book. **3b.** She will dial local phone numbers accurately. **3c.** She will engage in brief phone conversations with her daughters independently. **3d.** She will be able to request information or ask favors appropriately on the phone. **3e.** She will be able to take phone messages for her husband.
4. She will be able to prepare simple meals.	**4a.** She will name appliances in her kitchen, describe them, and demonstrate safe use. **4b.** She will state 4–5 steps needed to prepare simple meals. **4c.** She will be able to read labels and directions on food products.

individual's life based on an environmental needs assessment. Goals of this nature are listed in Appendix K. That list is not exhaustive, but suggests the communication skills needed in everyday activities. Some of the goals in Appendix K may have subgoals. Consideration, again, must be given to how performance will be judged and the possible stimulus, response, and environmental characteristics from Tables 3–15, 3–16, and 3–18.

Goals to address social competency are especially difficult to formulate. Liberman, DeRisi, and Mueser (1989) outline criteria for setting interpersonal goals as listed in Table 4–4. The first criterion is that goals should be stated in a positive, constructive manner. Second, as stressed throughout this book, goals should address behaviors that are of functional relevance to the individual. Behaviors that occur frequently and can be practiced often should be targeted, particularly at the beginning of treatment, to achieve early success with a behavior that is likely to have the greatest impact. Goals should be described in concrete, specific terms, including what the behavior is, when it is to occur, with whom, and where. A final criterion from Liberman, DeRisi, and Mueser (1989) is that the goal must be salient to the individual's current life situation.

The treatment plan segment shown in Table 4–3 is incomplete; additional columns are needed to indicate the methodology to be employed, persons responsible, and target completion dates for each goal.

General Treatment Strategies

One premise on which rehabilitation is built is that all individuals have the potential to learn. Injury to the brain affects learning, but almost all who recover from coma have the capacity for acquiring new behaviors (Giles & Clark-Wilson, 1993). The training techniques, however, must be carefully selected to match the individual's cognitive abilities and learning style. The more limited the learning abilities, the greater the need to rely on structuring of the environment and external supports and aids.

In general, the treatment strategies used traditionally by speech-language pathologists for retraining effective cognitive-linguistic abilities are a blend of information processing approaches from cognitive psychology (Adamovich et al., 1985) and behavior therapy approaches (Giles & Clark-Wilson, 1993; Goldstein et al., 1980; Jacobs, 1993; Liberman et al., 1989). In educational literature, similar treatment approaches have been called Direct Instruction (Engelmann & Carnine, 1982; Glang, Singer, Cooley, & Tish, 1992). Before detailing specific treatment strategies for rebuilding functional communication, general treatment approaches are outlined. These form the backbone of rehabilitation efforts and are the general treatment methods with which a clinician should operate to maximize learning potential.

Although the role of communication in social competence has been emphasized in this book, functional cognitive-communicative abilities go beyond this. Language and communication play a vital role in the mediation of cognition, behavior, and learning, as well as in social interactions (Carr & Durand, 1985; Gallagher, 1991; Wood, 1990). The speech-language pathologist must assist the rest of the team in establishing the effective use of language in all of these areas.

Table 4-4. Criteria for goals and examples of desirable and undesirable goal statements.

Criteria	Desirable Goal Statements	Undesirable Goal Statements
Positive and constructive	Ask job coach for help in an appropriate manner Maintain appropriate distance from communication partner	Stop talking back to supervisor Reduce inappropriate touching or hugging
Functional	Describe past work history in job interview Invite friend to go to movies	Express feelings to a therapist Ask for a favor of a therapist
High frequency	Initiate conversation with co-workers at lunch break Greet others when entering a room	Initiate conversation with co-workers at monthly meeting Express affection to spouse on birthday
Attainable	Maintain conversation for 2 minutes with friend Ask parents for permission to go to movies with friend	Maintain conversation with a stranger at the mall for 2 minutes Ask parents to buy a car
Specific	Generate three wh- questions during 2 minute conversation with friend Make phone calls to five apartment complexes and complete information sheet on each	Interact with others more often Locate an apartment
Current relevance	Use the phone to request refills of medication or set up Handi-Van transportation for work Explain abilities and past work history to prepare for upcoming job interview	Use the phone to inquire of opening and closing times at stores Express anger at previous boss for being laid off

Note: From *Social Skills Training for Psychiatric Patients* (p. 41) by R. P. Liberman, W. J. DeRisi, and K. T. Mueser, 1989, Needham Heights, MA: Allyn and Bacon. Copyright 1989 by Allyn and Bacon. Adapted by permission.

Clear, Consistent Instructions and Feedback

To be effective with individuals with learning needs, rehabilitation must be conducted in an environment in which communication is clear, logical, positive, unambiguous, and consistent (Giles & Clark-Wilson, 1993; Ylvisaker, Feeney, & Urbanczyk, 1993a, 1993b). That is, the purpose of the training and the rationale for training is clearly communicated. Treatment materials should be carefully organized, with clear expectations of performance explained to the individual. Giles and Clark-Wilson (1993) point out the need to highlight the essential elements of a task and the salient stimulus conditions to promote learning. A consistent approach to instructions and interactions should be maintained. Immediate feedback and reinforcement are used to provide explicit knowledge of the results or the quality of performance.

Hierarchical Organization

Skills should be taught in a hierarchical fashion, going from simple to more complex. Component skills are taught first, providing multiple opportunities for practicing a skill before moving to the next level or next skill area. Previous learning is highlighted and used to form a foundation to which new skills are attached. Periodic reviews consolidate learning and integrate new skills with old learning.

Training also moves from maximum structure during skill development to least structure necessary for successful maintenance in final stages. At the beginning, cueing, assistance, and external structure are used to build skills. As individuals demonstrate ability, they are gradually weaned, until the least structure necessary for continued success has been established.

Use of Strategies and Problem Solving

A processing and problem-solving approach should be taught to individuals, so that, if at all possible, they learn effective strategies for social interaction and learning, not just specific skills (Glang et al., 1992; Liberman et al., 1989; Ylvisaker et al., 1992). For example, training in perceiving and interpreting social information helps the individual determine what to do in future social situations. A problem-solving approach facilitates the generation and consideration of options for social interactions and correct decision making.

Use of Verbal Mediation

The use of verbal mediation in behavioral performance should be trained and reinforced, as well. Verbalization of an activity can assist in developing understanding of a task, in focusing attention on task elements and re quirements, in guiding the initiation and termination of behavior, and in regulating and inhibiting behavior (Giles & Clark-Wilson, 1993; Wood, 1990). All people tend to talk to themselves to learn a task or to guide themselves through a complex task. Although frontal lobe damage may disturb the ability of language to guide behavior (Luria, 1973), the efficacy of training overt verbal mediation, or "self-talk," has been demonstrated in a number of individuals with brain injuries and other populations (Malec, 1984; Stuss, Delgado, & Guzman, 1987).

Task Analysis

Task analysis is another key technique for clinicians to use when devising treatment protocols. This method involves analyzing and organizing complex tasks into components to make them easier to learn. This can be used to help individuals perform a task in an organized manner, to train for component mastery, so that they can be chained together to perform an entire task, to develop checklists for external reminders for completion of a task, or to develop systematic assessment procedures for functional tasks. Use of task analysis is presented again in the next chapter.

Positive, "Anything That Works" Attitude

Clinicians need to maintain a positive, problem solving approach to treatment, themselves. Individuals in treatment must be treated with respect, in an age-appropriate manner, and in a manner that facilitates competence in their environment. If an individual is displaying inappropriate behavior or is not successful at a task, the clinician should reexamine the approach, strategies, or task involved to determine the underlying breakdown. Failures at a therapy task often indicate that the clinician has used the wrong approach. People generally try to do the best they can with their abilities. When the response to a task is wrong or unusual, the clinician should try to "get inside the individual's head," speculate on why the person performed in that manner, and then assist the individual in developing a more effective strategy. As stated by Willer (1993), rehabilitation should be practical yet "use whatever it takes to accomplish the goal of community reintegration" (p. 6).

Use of Natural Consequences

It is important, however, that individuals with brain injury be permitted to experience the natural consequences of their effective and ineffective communication or behaviors. Opportunities for decision making, control over events in their environment, and personal responsibility must be integrated into the treatment. The clinician's role should be viewed more as that of an advisor, coach, mentor, and facilitator in enhancing an individual's sense of self-control and determination. The perception of control and a feeling of competency are critical for the motivation to continue to work on mastery of a skill (McCombs, 1988).

Techniques That Facilitate Behavioral Learning

A number of associative learning, or behavioral therapy, techniques are typically used to train or retrain functional cognitive-communication abilities (Giles & Clark-Wilson, 1993; Liberman et al., 1989). These can be used in training social communication, functional daily living activities, or use of compensatory strategies. Some of the most widely used methods are listed in Table 4–5 and described below.

Setting Positive Expectations and Using Goal Statements

An individual's personal goals should be reviewed at the beginning of each treatment session and tied into the expectations of the intervention. This provides consistency to treatment, facilitates understanding of the relevance of a task, and highlights what is to be learned.

Direct Instructions and Scripting

This consists of providing the individual with detailed information concerning the desired behavior. For example, types and examples of nonverbal communication behaviors and their use in social situations can be discussed and demonstrated. Then a script is provided for the individual to follow to practice the expected behavioral response in a given situation.

Modeling and Imitation

Appropriate and effective behavior is modeled for the individual to imitate. A model of inappropriate behavior also may be provided to heighten

Table 4–5. Techniques that facilitate behavioral learning.

Setting positive expectations and using goal statements

Direct instructions and scripting

Modeling and imitation

Behavioral rehearsal

Role playing

Shaping

Cueing and fading of cueing

Videotaped feedback

Corrective feedback from peers and therapists

Social reinforcement

an individual's ability to recognize the desired behavioral response and understand the importance of effective communication behavior.

Behavioral Rehearsal

Opportunities are provided for the individual to practice a desired behavior. In this way, the individual can try alternative approaches to the situation or alternative wordings. A rehearsal may be subvocal or a "dry-run" to a role play situation.

Role Playing

Through simulation of real-life events, the individual has an opportunity in a supportive environment to practice skills that are socially relevant.

Shaping

When an individual is initially not capable of producing a desired behavior, close approximations are reinforced. The criterion for reinforcement is gradually increased until mastery is achieved. For example, an individual may not initially be able to generate questions to maintain a conversation. The individual is instructed to just attend to a partner and nod and is reinforced for this behavior. Later, the person's goal is to ask just one question and eventually to engage in more equal conversational turn taking.

Cueing and Fading of Cues

Cues or prompts can be verbal or nonverbal, written or oral, specific or nonspecific, as outlined in Chapter 3. Initially, extensive cueing should be used to ensure adequate performance. Cueing should be faded gradually so that the individual depends less and less on environmental cues. Fading of cues can be conducted by delaying the prompting or through use of less direct (verbal versus physical) or less specific cues (e.g., What comes next?) (Giles & Clark-Wilson, 1993).

Feedback Designed to Build Self-Evaluation and Self-Monitoring

Various forms of feedback should be incorporated in training, including videotape, peer, and therapist to furnish knowledge of performance. Videotape feedback allows the clinician to explicitly identify effective or ineffective features of an interaction. The individual is able to look back at his or her performance and become aware of strengths and weaknesses.

It is critical to include time for self-evaluation. Ben-Yishay and Lakin (1989) start feedback after a group exercise with an individual who is "in the hot seat." The individual is coached on evaluating his or her performance, based on the set criteria for the exercise.

Corrective feedback from peers and staff is another important method. It must be structured so that it is concrete, concise, and related back to the stated goals and expectations for the individual. Negative personal statements should be avoided; rather individuals should be told what they did well and what they could have improved, with specific means for improving performance given.

Social Reinforcement

Positive and effective social behaviors should be reinforced by the therapist through use of praise, attention, or recognition. The therapist can encourage others in the environment to reward appropriate communicative behavior.

Promoting Maintenance, Transfer, and Generalization

As stated in the first chapter, one of the major challenges to successful community reintegration is the problem of maintenance of skills over time, transfer of learning to related tasks or settings, and generalization of skills and learning to other contexts, especially to the discharge environment (Cicerone & Tupper, 1986; Durgin, Cullity, & Devine, 1991; Wilson, 1987). To overcome these obstacles, thought must be given at the very beginning of treatment, not at the end. Activities and techniques that promote generalization should be an integral part of a treatment program (Durgin et al., 1991; Liberman et al., 1989; McReynolds, 1989; Stokes & Baer, 1977; Thompson, 1989; Ylvisaker, Urbanczyk, & Feeney, 1992).

As stated before, maintaining a functional approach to treatment and keeping in mind the principles of treatment listed at the beginning of this chapter help promote generalization. Table 4–6 summarizes specific techniques that have been found to foster generalization, maintenance, and transfer of learning.

A primary consideration is the selection of behaviors for training (Thompson, 1989; Liberman et al., 1989). Therapy should target those behaviors that are functionally relevant to the natural environment or structurally related to responses the person needs to succeed in natural settings. This is a restatement of the third and fourth principles from Table 4–1. For example, instead of working to improve vocabulary for the sake of improving vocabulary, the goal should be to improve comprehension and expression of names of tools needed on a job or terms needed for banking. Success at these tasks would receive natural reinforcement (e.g., selection of appropriate tool to accomplish a task at work, successfully cashing a check) and facilitate maintenance and generalization.

The use of multiple stimulus exemplars in multiple settings with a variety of persons also promotes generalization (McReynolds, 1989; Stokes & Baer, 1977; Thompson, 1989). If possible, settings that are similar to natural environments and practice with persons of similar characteristics to those in

Table 4-6.   Strategies that promote maintenance and generalization of skills.

Reducing differences between treatment and natural conditions

Training with multiple and/or relevant persons

Training in multiple settings

Use of natural reinforcers

Training significant others to deliver reinforcement

Overlearning

Training in self-monitoring strategies

Training in self-reinforcement

In *vivo* coaching

Homework assignments

Regular booster sessions after treatment

natural settings are preferable. The use of natural reinforcers, that is, obtaining material needs or needed information and social acceptance, should be incorporated into the training procedures.

Inclusion of the family in the rehabilitation process is important for a number of reasons, but particularly to assist in the transfer and generalization of skills to natural environments (Liberman et al., 1989; Ylvisaker et al., 1992). To facilitate stabilization and generalization of a desired behavior, the family should be trained in specific behavioral expectations for their loved one. They need to know to reinforce desirable behaviors and to not accept behaviors that are less than what the person is capable of performing. For example, the team may have set a goal for an individual to speak with adequate loudness rather than "mumbling." The individual is trained to discriminate an acceptable loudness level from an inappropriately soft level. Team members cue the individual at first and then ignore the individual unless the appropriate loudness level is used. The family, on the other hand, continues to give the person attention, getting closer to the individual, putting their arms around the person, and asking for repetition when there is mumbling. The behavior will not change or the change will not be enduring if the family is not made a part of the treatment team, extending training to their interactions with the individual. It may be important for the family to be included in treatment sessions with the individual.

Repetition of the target behavior beyond achievement of initial success or overlearning of a behavior helps to make the behavior more automatic. This increases the likelihood that it will be maintained over time and will occur in other situations. Overpractice ensures that a target behavior has been established as a habit pattern.

The importance of incorporating self-monitoring procedures for generalization to natural environments also has been demonstrated (Durgin et al., 1991; Koegel, Koegel, & Ingram, 1986; Schloss, Thompson, Gajar, & Schloss, 1985). This strategy increases the active participation of an individual in the treatment program. The individual is trained to recognize the occurrence of the target behavior and to record that occurrence.

Individuals also should be taught self-reinforcement as a means of maintaining effective communication behavior within the self-monitoring program. In other words, individuals should be trained to use positive self-statements, such as, "I handled that situation really well" or "Good job, Frank, for completing the instructions you were given."

In vivo training is another strategy for promoting maintenance and generalization of skills. Prompting, reinforcement, shaping, fading, and other behavioral procedures are used in socially relevant settings, such as an individual's home or a restaurant, to teach a skill (Wong et al., 1993; Ylvisaker et al., 1992). Although limited investigation has yet occurred, the coaching of appropriate social skills in natural settings has been found to be an effective method for persons with schizophrenia (Wong et al., 1993; Wong & Woolsey, 1989). It has the advantage of directly promoting success in the natural setting. Lennox and Brune (1993) report a successful single case study of the use of training in natural, unstructured interactions in a home environment with an individual with severe communication problems.

Developing a problem-solving approach to social interactions is another technique felt to enhance generalization (Liberman et al., 1989). Because it is impossible to teach a person all the specific social skills needed in the real world, it is best to provide strategies for generating alternatives and solutions to interpersonal challenges (Liberman et al., 1989; Ylvisaker et al., 1992).

Additional strategies are the use of homework assignments and provision of follow-up services or booster sessions. The latter is an important aspect but rarely fully addressed in many rehabilitation programs.

Group Treatment Considerations

One decision regarding intervention is on the use of individual or group treatment as best meeting the needs of an individual. At the beginning of intervention, a clinician may need individual time to establish the personal communication goals, to develop and implement specific internal compensatory strategies or external aids, or to rebuild underlying speech, cognitive, and language skills. When the clinician is providing treatment within an individual's home, the treatment, of course, will be conducted on an individual basis.

For individuals at the postacute stage of rehabilitation, however, group therapy offers many benefits (Deaton, 1991; Sohlberg & Mateer, 1989b). It provides an opportunity to observe and practice social communication skills in a more natural context. In many instances, the functional limitations of the individual are more apparent in group situations than in one-on-one settings.

Groups also may provide opportunities for individuals to obtain valuable feedback and support from multiple sources, especially peers. Feedback from peers is important for developing better self-awareness of strengths and needs, a frequent issue for persons with brain injury, and greater acceptance of current functional abilities. Groups provide opportunities for individuals to learn from peers through observation and modeling, as opposed to working with a therapist, alone. In addition, because the interactants are peers rather than therapists, skills are more likely to generalize to other settings.

Groups also may help individuals to build relationships and lead to a stronger sense of social support. Groups help prepare individuals for resuming social roles and permit them to try new cognitive-communicative skills in social situations (Hill & Carper, 1985). Groups permit the targeting and practicing of positive psychosocial interactions. This may be more motivating for many clients than working on goals individually.

Group treatment has the obvious cost benefit over individual treatment in terms of personnel and financial considerations. The clinician must ensure, however, that groups are tailored to meet the needs of individuals. Groups may not be appropriate for all individuals.

Group size is an important consideration. As the number of members increase, the time for each to participate decreases, and it may become increasingly difficult for individuals to feel comfortable in speaking (Sampson & Marthas, 1990). On the other hand, very small groups of only two or three members offer less diversity of resources for problem solving. Liberman et al. (1989) advocate a size of 6 to 10 individuals in social skills training groups. Considerations in determining size include the specific needs of the individuals, the severity of their needs, and the availability of a co-leader.

Leadership of Group Treatment

Leading group therapy is very demanding, both from a cognitive and an interpersonal perspective, especially with individuals with brain injury. It is important that a leader of group treatment be prepared for the responsibility. As stated in Sohlberg and Mateer (1989b), the behaviors of group members must immediately be evaluated and responded to. To promote the group process, the leader must provide support, structure, and feedback, yet stay out of the immediate focus. As Deaton (1991) points out, individuals with brain injury in a group session may appear unmotivated, apathetic, irritated, or even hostile. The leader must be flexible, enthusiastic, and capable of handling behavioral challenges.

Corrective Feedback by Group Leader

Sampson and Marthas (1990) discuss the role of a group leader in helping individuals process information and providing corrective feedback on interpersonal skills. They offer the model shown in Table 4–7 for a group leader providing feedback.

The model is put into action by:

1. What did I see? Feedback is provided in a concrete manner relating to the behavior that was observed, such as use of a harsh tone of voice or the lack of eye contact.

2. How does it affect me? The feedback describes the effect of a given behavior on the leader and the general interpretation of that behavior. For example, "I felt that your voice was loud and harsh. When you speak that way people will think you're angry if you speak loudly and avoid talking with you.

3. Is this perception and its effects shared by others? The leader's observations and conclusions are checked against those of other members of the group, by asking if others feel the same way.

4. What can be done about it? The leader opens the floor for discussion of how to improve the interaction.

Ben-Yishay uses the "sandwich technique" for providing corrective feedback to individuals (cited in Prigatano, 1989). A positive statement about the individual is given first, then the negative feedback is given, and a positive note is used in the closing. An example of this would be:

Jane, you have made gains in paying attention to the person speaking. However, when you respond in such an angry-sounding voice, others become frightened or angry. If you think about what to say first and then say it in a more pleasant voice, others will see you as more competent and are more likely to really listen to you. I know you have the ability to do this. Jane, I want to thank you for having the maturity to listen to what I had to say.

Table 4–7.   Suggested model for feedback given by a leader to a group member.

---

1. What did I see?

2. How does it affect me?

3. Is this perception and its effects shared by others?

4. What can be done about it?

Note: From *Group Process for the Health Professions* (3rd ed.) (p. 204) by E. E. Sampson and M. Marthas, 1990, Albany, NY: Delmar Publishers. Copyright 1990 by Delmar Publishers, Inc. Reproduced by permission.

Intervention Techniques of Group Leaders

Ten specific intervention techniques to be used by group leaders, outlined by Sampson and Marthas (1990), are shown in Table 4–8. *Support* should be provided to let the group members know they are on track, to promote group trust, and to create a climate of acceptance in which even unpopular responses or feedback can be given. *Confrontation* by the leader offers a challenge to an individual to examine his or her behavior from another perspective. *Advice, information,* and *suggestions* may be offered, based on the leader's expertise and knowledge.

As listed in Table 4–8, the leader also helps to keep the group proceding in an organized and focused manner in many ways. One way to maintain the focus on important issues, reach consensus, and organize information is by *summarizing* what has happened and setting the agenda for the next session. *Probing* and *questioning* can be used to help group members elaborate on ideas that might have been left incomplete and to facilitate complete exploration of ideas. Through *clarification,* the leader can reduce miscommunication and key in on important concepts. *Repetition, paraphrasing,* and *highlighting* are additional techniques for inviting expansion of ideas, for spotlighting important points, and for sharpening members' understanding of what has been said.

The leader can offer *reflection of feelings,* or facilitate the understanding of feelings that may underlie what is said or done. With *reflection of behaviors,* the leader can help members understand how their behavior is perceived by others and the consequences of these perceptions. The leader can offer an *interpretation* and *analysis* of situations regarding themes and patterns of behavior as well as the underlying meanings. Finally, the leader must model and encourage *listening,* an important aspect of social interaction, to help others understand the importance of shared communication and concern.

The leader is responsible for generating specific goals and objectives to be accomplished within the group and goals for each individual that can be accomplished through the group setting. An agenda that each session will follow should be established by the leader. The leader also should facilitate the group's development of rules for participation (Sohlberg & Mateer, 1989b). Different types of groups used in the rehabilitation of persons with brain injuries and the objectives are described in Deaton (1991), Hill and Carper (1985), and Sohlberg and Mateer (1989b). Specific techniques for improving communication through group treatment will be covered in the next chapter.

Sequence of Intervention Focus

When weighing evaluation results and multiple needs for intervention, it is helpful to have a guideline for sequencing treatment needs and the various intervention models. Several leaders in brain injury rehabilitation

Table 4–8. Interventions provided by group leaders.

Intervention	Purpose
Support	Provides supportive climate for expressing ideas and opinions, including unpopular or unusual points of view. Facilitates members continuing with their ongoing behavior. Helps reinforce positive forms of behavior. Creates a climate in which silent members may feel secure enough to participate.
Confrontation	Aids in growth and development; helps unfreeze members from being stuck in one mode of functioning. Helps reduce some forms of disruptive behavior. Helps members deal more openly and directly with each other.
Advice and Suggestions	Shares expertise, offers new perspectives.
Summarizing	Helps keep group on its task by reviewing past actions and by setting agenda for future sessions. Brings to focus still unresolved issues. Organizes past in ways that help clarify; brings into focus themes and patterns of interaction.
Clarifying	Helps reduce distortion in communication. Facilitates focus on substantive issues rather than allowing members to be sidetracked into misunderstandings.
Probing and Questioning	Helps expand a point that may have been left incomplete. Gets at more extensive and wider range of information. Invites members to explore their ideas in greater detail.
Repeating, Paraphrasing, and Highlighting	Helps members continue with their ongoing behavior; invites further exploration and examination of what is being said. Clarifies and helps focus on the specific, important, or key aspect of a communication. Sharpens members' understanding of what is being said or done.
Reflecting: Feelings	Orients members to the feelings that may lie behind what is being said or done. Helps members deal with issues they might otherwise avoid or miss.

Intervention	Purpose
Reflecting: Behavior	Gives members the opportunity to see how their behavior appears to others and to see and evaluate its consequences.
	Helps members to understand others' perceptions and responses to them.
Interpretation and Analysis	Renders behavior meaningful by locating it in a larger context in which a causal explanation is provided.
Listening	Provides an attentive and responsive audience for those who participate.
	Models a helpful way for members to relate to one another; gives a feeling of sharing and mutual concern.
	Helps members sharpen their own ideas and thinking as they realize that indeed others are listening and concerned about what they are saying.

Note: From *Group Process for the Health Professions* (3rd ed.) (pp. 222–224) by E. E. Sampson and M. Marthas, 1990, Albany, NY: Delmar Publishers. Copyright 1990 by Delmar Publishers, Inc. Reproduced by permission.

have provided frameworks for a hierarchy of treatment that promote community reintegration.

Malkmus (1989) suggested a sequence of priorities in cognitive-communicative goals to lead to effective social communication in everyday settings. As shown in Table 4–9, the first point of focus in Malkmus' framework is to reestablish the underlying cognitive and language components of social communication. This step is particularly important for individuals who continue to have significant cognitive and language deficits that preclude establishment of functional skills. From the beginning and all along the way, however, compensatory strategies and environmental adaptations should be developed and implemented to overcome persisting cognitive and communicative impairments.

As quickly as possible, the focus should move to reestablishing social skills or communicative competence, Malkmus (1989) states. Training should turn to addressing conversational abilities that will enable the individual to achieve both material and relationship needs. The focus would next shift to building and reinforcing problem-solving and self-regulatory behaviors that are necessary for skilled psychosocial behavior and social adaptation. The final step is to integrate these acquired social behaviors into real-life contexts.

Table 4–9.   Sequence of treatment suggested by Malkmus (1989).

Rebuilding underlying cognitive and language components

Developing compensatory strategies and modifying environment

Rebuilding communicative competence

Rebuilding skilled social behavior

Application of skills into real-world settings

Ben-Yishay and colleagues (Ben-Yishay & Lakin, 1989) also provide a hierarchical model for brain injury rehabilitation. As shown in Figure 4–1, rehabilitation should first focus on getting individuals to be actively engaged in their rehabilitation and to be open or malleable to rehabilitation. During this stage, individuals are helped to understand their deficits and to accept coaching from others and the use of compensatory methods. Care is taken not to decrease the individual's will to overcome the deficits, but acceptance of realistic goals and outcomes is emphasized. To assist individuals in being actively engaged in rehabilitation, they are taught early on how to focus their attention, sustain concentration, and reflect on their own behavior. The importance of initiating and controlling their behavior is also addressed at this level.

The next step in Ben-Yishay's model is to build compensation for the deficits and mastery over life scripts and therapy tasks. The individuals' residual abilities and learning capacities are identified. Problem solving and self-monitoring are trained as compensatory strategies, first in therapy exercises and then in functional tasks.

As an individual begins to make changes and adjustments and use the compensatory strategies and skills in functional settings, increased competence is attained. Increased productivity and self-sufficiency in community, work, and family situations help individuals adjust better and thus lead to greater acceptance of their situation and an increased sense of self-identity.

Summary

This chapter has identified key principles and methods of goal setting and intervention for a functional approach to rehabilitation of cognitive-communication abilities. Treatment planning must start with the identification of the desired long-term goals through a process, such as Futures Planning. Based on results of the process, appropriate intermediate and short-term goals can be set. Two lists of functional goals were provided as examples, as well as criteria for establishing interpersonal goals. The various models and methods of intervention were reviewed, highlighting techniques that promote the transfer and generalization of skills.

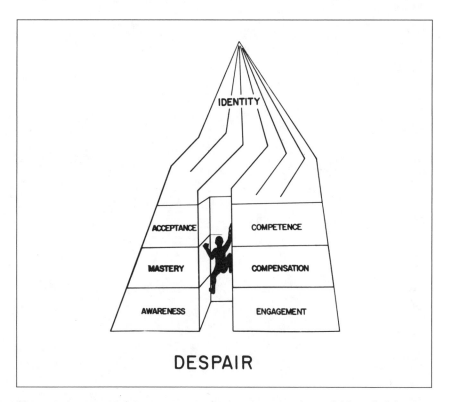

Figure 4-1. New York University Head Trauma Program's model for rehabilitation following brain injury. *Note*: From "Structured Group Treatment for Brain-Injury Survivors" (p. 292) by Y. Ben-Yishay and P. Lakin, 1989. In D. W. Ellis and A-L Christensen (Eds.), *Neuropsychological Treatment After Brain Injury*. Boston: Kluwer Academic Publishers. Copyright 1989 by Kluwer Academic Publishers. Reprinted by permission.

The clinician must decide on the most appropriate format of treatment in terms of individual versus group sessions. Consideration also must be given to the sequence of priorities in treatment. Foremost must be the objective of increasing community participation and options for community integration for an individual. The next chapter provides more detail on specific intervention strategies to build communicative competence.

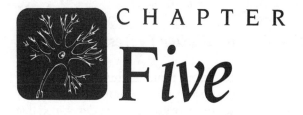

CHAPTER

Five

Rebuilding Cognitive-Communicative Competence and Community Integration

Based on the groundwork of treatment planning and goal setting, this chapter provides greater detail on intervention strategies for rebuilding communicative competence and achieving social and community reintegration. Consideration will be given to each of the models of intervention that are appropriate in postacute rehabilitation in the sequence proposed by Malkmus (1989) and to the components in the model of communicative competence presented in Chapter 2 (Figure 2–1). That is, strategies that address the first priorities in treatment—to ensure adequate functioning in cognitive-communicative processes, teach applicable compensatory strategies, and provide appropriate environmental adaptations—are addressed first. Considered next are techniques that address other components of the model that build communicative competence directly as well as develop higher-level reasoning, problem solving, coping, and decision-making abilities. Finally, ideas for improving the integration of skills into community situations are presented.

Rebuilding Cognitive-Communicative Processes

In the early days of cognitive rehabilitation, much enthusiasm and effort were devoted to drills designed to improve a specific cognitive process. Many computer software programs and cognitive workbooks were developed that included reaction time, visual perceptual, attention, or memory drills. The belief was that, through multiple and repeated experiences, the impaired component would be "repaired." Though a place still exists for this model of intervention, it is generally agreed that focusing on retraining cognitive-linguistic component processes, alone, is ineffective in achieving community reintegration goals (Gordon & Hibbard, 1991; Wood, 1990; Ylvisaker & Urbanczyk, 1990). Even though individuals may improve on the computer drill or the task that is used, there is limited evidence that these exercises lead to improvement in untrained tasks or in functional activities.

Benefit may be derived from component cognitive process training when the goal is to create an awareness of strengths or weaknesses, to develop strategies to improve cognitive-linguistic functions, or to demonstrate the efficacy of a compensatory strategy. Computer-based training offers the advantage of providing rapid feedback of performance. By contrasting performance without and with use of a compensatory strategy, such as verbal repetition, the clinician can demonstrate the effectiveness of strategies to overcome deficits. Computer tasks offer the additional advantage that many individuals are highly motivated to perform them.

Attention-Specific Training

Some evidence suggests that attention may be amenable to improvement through specific training (for review of studies in this area, see Ruff, Niemann, Troster, & Mateer, 1990). Attentional processes are critical, because they form the foundation for all other cognitive processes—for accurate information processing, for storage of information, and for communicative competence (Mateer & Sohlberg, 1992). Therefore, improvement in this area theoretically would have major significance in functional life activities.

Ben-Yishay and his colleagues at the New York University Medical Center (Ben-Yishay & Diller, 1983; Ben-Yishay, Piasetsky, & Rattock, 1987; Ben-Yishay, Rattok, & Diller, 1979) were the first to suggest that attentional processes could be improved through a process-specific training program. Tasks used in their training program were designed primarily to improve vigilance, reaction time, and anticipatory set. The degree of carryover to functional tasks was noted to vary from individual to individual (Ben-Yishay et al., 1987).

Sohlberg and Mateer (1987) developed an attentional treatment program called Attention Process Training (APT) and demonstrated its effectiveness with both mildly as well as severely injured individuals (Mateer & Sohlberg, 1988; Mateer, Sohlberg, & Youngman, 1990). APT consists of a set of hierarchically organized training procedures designed to improve focused, sustained, selective, alternating, and divided attention. Mateer and Sohlberg (1992), however, indicate that severely injured individuals require additional training to generalize improved attentional skills to functional settings and that attentional process training is ineffective for some individuals.

In two other studies of the efficacy of process-specific training in attention, Wood and Fussey (1987) and Ponsford and Kinsella (1988), improvement was found on specific tasks, but little effect was seen in more natural tasks. These researchers did, however, find that the behavioral aspects of attention—sitting and paying attention and maintaining alertness to a task—improved with feedback and reinforcement.

One way to maintain a functional approach to working on component processes is to target the process or skill in functional tasks. For example, attention to task is an important work skill. Therefore, feedback and reinforcement as well as other behavioral techniques can be used to increase an individual's attention while performing a specific functional task (Giles & Clark-Wilson, 1993). The individual might receive praise for paying attention when sorting mail for increasing lengths of time and be shown a graph that demonstrates this or other data, such as increased speed in sorting. Other examples of functional attention tasks include attending to spoken paragraphs of increasing length or attending to a group discussion for an increasing length of time.

Memory Retraining

Most of the cognitive remediation software or workbook tasks designed to improve memory consist of repetitive practice at recalling lists of letters, digits, words, sentences, shapes, or patterns. The problem with these tasks is that they do not resemble natural memory tasks and there is little evidence that demonstrates their efficacy. In part, this is because these tasks target the attentional-based encoding aspects of memory but not the storage or retrieval aspects (Ruff et al., 1990).

One approach to memory retraining is Prospective Memory Training (PMT) developed by Mateer and Sohlberg (1988, 1992). Prospective memory is defined as "the ability to remember to carry out specified actions at future target times" (1992, p. 286). Rehabilitation in this area has great functional significance, because this is the type of memory often required in everyday situations and prospective memory failures are the most frequently experienced type of memory failures reported by individuals with brain injuries (Mateer, Sohlberg, & Crinean, 1987). The goal of PMT is to progressively extend in a step-by-step manner the length of time an individual is able to remember to carry out a specific verbal command. The efficacy of this approach was demonstrated by single-case studies in Sohlberg, White, Evans, and Mateer (1992a, 1992b).

Another example of a functional approach to memory retraining is that of Schacter and Glisky (1986). Their approach was to teach the individual domain-specific knowledge, "knowledge pertaining to a particular task, subject, or function that is important to a patient in his or her everyday life" (p. 265). Treatment tasks simulate what the individual will encounter in real-life living, social, or work activities. Examples include training of names of co-workers or close friends, facts needed to succeed in a course or on the job, or a particular work skill or task. Schacter and Glisky (1986) demonstrated that even severely amnesic individuals can be taught specific information and skills. Their results indicate that use of vanishing cues is superior to simple repetition for teaching vocabulary. In this method, the individual must complete part of a new vocabulary word each trial, with the fragment cue being reduced gradually across trials.

Personal Compensatory Strategy Training

The training of general and specific personal compensatory strategies is an important functional approach to cognitive-communication intervention. A personal compensatory strategy is defined as "a deliberate, self-initiated application of a procedure to achieve a goal that is difficult to achieve because of impaired functioning" (Szekeres et al., 1985, p. 237). This approach makes use of strengths and preserved skills to overcome the challenges caused by brain injury.

Personal compensatory strategies can be either *overt*, or *external aids* (such as a memory notebook), or *covert*, or *internal strategies* (such as subvocal repetition of a phone number to remember it) (Szekeres et al., 1985). As Milton and Wertz (1986) point out, "an effective strategy uses what a patient can do to assist in compensating for what cannot be done" (p. 244). For example, an individual may not be able to remember the phone numbers of relatives, but can read. A list of phone numbers, then, can be written and placed by the phone or in the wallet for reference when needed.

Most personal compensatory strategies are ways to provide structure and consistency for an individual to compensate for problems in memory, planning, initiation, or organization. The types of strategies that can be used are limited only by a clinician's creativity. The clinician must use the assessment information regarding cognitive-communicative strengths and needs to tailor the management strategies so that an individual is able to accomplish everyday activities.

The individual's communication skills should be kept in mind as the strategies are developed (Milton, 1985). For example, writing information down will not be an effective way to compensate for memory challenges for a person who cannot read or one who cannot produce legible writing. Either the underlying communication skills must be retrained first or alternative approaches, such as use of pictures or word lists from which selection is made, must be considered.

It is important that an individual be involved in the development of personal strategies to assure acceptance of selected methods (Milton, 1985; Milton & Wertz, 1986). If an individual has been noted to use compensatory strategies in certain instances, treatment can begin by refining these strategies. At times, when compliance is an issue and when no health or safety risks are involved, it may be necessary to let individuals try to perform a task without a method of compensation for a problem, such as buying groceries and let them suffer the natual consequences. If the individual forgets to buy ground beef for dinner, then he or she must either return to the store or change the menu. Another way to facilitate compliance is to demonstrate the effectiveness of compensatory strategies, as already discussed, through computer-based cognitive exercises with and without use of a compensatory strategy.

The strategies must be modeled and reinforced in appropriate real-life situations, whenever possible, to ensure use outside the clinical setting (Hart & Hayden, 1986). Training should develop the use of the strategy until it is established in procedural memory. Examples and lists of internal and external strategies for compensating for cognitive-communicative deficits can be found in Haarbauer-Krupa, Henry et al. (1985); Milton (1985, 1988); Milton and Wertz (1986); and Ylvisaker and Gobble (1987).

Milton (1985) identified a number of general areas for which she found training in use of compensatory strategies to increase competency in everyday life:

1. Knowing what to do
2. Time management
3. Organization and retrieval of information
4. Community mobility
5. Household management
6. Using the telephone

Many different types of internal and external personal compensatory strategies exist. A number are now discussed.

Internal Compensatory Strategies

Internal strategies use internally generated methods for improving perform-ance. As Giles and Clark-Wilson (1993) point out, everyone uses in-ternal strategies to facilitate information processing. Many internal strate-gies rely on verbal mediation, attempting to develop greater self-regulation of cognitive processing and behavior. For example, when someone's name cannot be retrieved, a person may self-cue by going through the alphabet. One strategy used for improving attention after brain injury is to train an individual to use self-instructions such as, "Pay attention," or self-ques-tions such as, "What am I supposed to be doing now?" (Haarbauer-Krupa, Henry et al., 1985). Other strategies are attempts by an individual to gain control of environmental, or input, factors. For example, an individual can request information from others when a memory failure occurs or can ask for a speaker to repeat information when slowed processing interferes with comprehension.

Memory retraining has often focused on teaching a variety of internal strategies (Parenté & DiCesare, 1991; Wilson, 1987). Visual imagery, mnemonic strategies, and verbal rehearsal are the most commonly used internal compensatory strategies for memory challenges. Other strategies include verbal labeling and chunking (grouping) of information (Parenté & DiCesare, 1991). Although many of these strategies do facilitate performance on a particular task, individuals with TBI (as well as non-disabled individuals) often fail to use the strategies spontaneously (Press-ley, 1993).

These strategies may be valuable, however, in teaching context specific information, such as information needed on the job or in school (Parenté & Anderson-Parenté, 1989, 1990). A clinician can help an individual develop a rhyme or acronym to remember such information.

Training in use of internal strategies is one of the major approaches to rehabilitation of executive or metacognitive dysfunction. Employment of internal strategies, however, requires that an indiviual is aware that there is a need for compensation. The first step may need to be training in self-awareness (see Barco, Crosson, Bolesta, Werts, & Stout, 1991; Crosson et al., 1989). As Ylvisaker and Szekeres (1989) state, "patients need to know what they can do well and what they cannot do well in relation to their goals" (p. 43). The writers suggest balancing confrontational feedback with self-discovery. Use of a series of tasks is recommended, so that a clinician can help an individual isolate factors that interfere with the per-formance of a task and identify strategies that can improve performance. The individual is asked for his or her ideas for improving performance and to critically evaluate the results.

"Self-talk," or verbal self-regulation, training programs have been found to be useful for some individuals after brain injury (Burgess &

Alderman, 1987; Cicerone & Wood, 1987; Lawson & Rice, 1989; Webster & Scott, 1983). These programs generally train an individual to use initially overt and later covert self-statements for analyzing tasks, selecting and intiating strategies, and self-monitoring during performance. Cicerone and Giacino (1992) report a case of improved performance when an individual received specific training in error recognition and error utilization.

Training in self-monitoring of conversational behaviors is a critical part of building communicative competence. Gajar, Schloss, Schloss, and Thompson (1984) and Schloss, Thompson, Gajar, and Schloss (1985) demonstrate that training in self-monitoring can lead to improved conversational skills in both structured and natural situations. In addition, the results were found to be maintained over at least a month posttreatment (Schloss et al., 1985). The conversational behaviors targeted included self-disclosure, topic maintenance, interruptions, and inappropriate laughter. Training in self-monitoring has also been found to reduce dysfluencies in persons with mild aphasia (Whitney & Goldstein, 1989).

Training in use of cognitive strategies can improve performance as long as there is an external prompt, such as from a clinician, to use a strategy. The challenge lies in getting an individual to continue to use a strategy and to recognize when and where to apply it (Pressley, 1993). Impulsivity, anxiety, and indifference all interfere with strategy application and success (Pressley, 1993; Ylvisaker, 1992).

Additional information on internal strategies, especially self-management, is presented later in this chapter.

External Compensatory Strategies

External compensatory strategies can take many forms. Most are low-tech involving the use of paper and pencil. Others employ high-tech electronics. Commonly used external aids include the following.

Checklists, Schedules, and Planning Aids

Many very important compensatory strategies are in the form of written (or pictorial) checklists, schedules, or planning aids. Through a task analysis, a clinician determines the specific steps involved in completing a given task, along with the materials for completing the task. A written checklist or form is then devised to assist the individual in sequencing, organizing, and completing the task. Checklists tailored to the needs of a particular individual often are necessary before the individual can independently complete all morning activities of daily living and remember to take items needed for the rest of the day. Figure 5–1 is an example of a morning checklist for a young man who lived in a supervised apartment and had a volunteer work position.

Morning Checklist

_____   Take a shower

_____   Shave (check left side carefully)

_____   Get dressed (wear clean sports shirt with nice pants for work)

_____   Brush hair

_____   Eat breakfast

_____   Brush teeth

_____   Clean glasses, if needed

_____   Get all items needed:

        _____   Wallet

        _____   Change for bus

        _____   Glasses

        _____   Memory notebook

        _____   Lunch

        _____   Apartment key

Be out the door by 7:30!

Figure 5–1. Example of a morning checklist used in a supervised apartment with an individual with severe memory challenges.

The checklist is placed in a prominent place as a cue to the individual to perform each step or task and then to place a mark in the proper place. At first, training is often needed for effective use of a checklist. Some individuals are able to learn a routine to the point that the checklist becomes unnecessary. However, the behavior should be extremely stable before weaning the individual from the checklist.

Planning aids can be developed for any particular activity or to assist in general planning and execution of a task. Gobble, Henry, Pfahl, and Smith (1987) developed an excellent task analysis, or "structured thinking" form, shown in Figure 5–2, to help individuals organize, plan, and monitor specific work assignments. Planning forms can also be devised to assist in planning and executing a leisure or community outing. An example of such a form, developed at the author's facility, is shown in Figure 5–3. Other examples of community outing planning forms can be found in Cullity, Jackson, and Shaw (1991) and Milton (1985).

Additional examples of these types of checklists and planning aids for assistance in daily living and vocational activities are in Condeluci, Cooperman, and Seif (1987); Kreutzer, Wehman, Morton, and Stonnington (1988); Milton (1985); and Milton and Wertz (1986).

1. Task: Directions/Notes   **Materials Needed:**

- Are there time limits?
- Do I understand what I'm to do?
- Do I have all the information I need?

2. Plan

Steps:

3. Review

- Are my steps and materials accurate?

Yes   No

Rethink steps and materials

Ask for additional information if necessary

DO IT

4. Final Evaluation

- Does my work look acceptable?
- Is it done on time?
- Any special concerns:

Figure 5–2. Structured thinking form. *Note*: From "Work Adjustment Services" (p. 239) by E. M. Gobble, K. Henry, J. Knight, and G. Smith, 1987. In M. Ylvisaker and E. M. Gobble (Eds.), *Community Re-Entry for Head Injured Adults*, Austin, TX: Pro-Ed. Copyright 1987 by Pro-Ed. Reprinted by permission.

Simple Maps

For individuals with problems in visuospatial orientation or memory, simple maps may help them locate offices within the rehabilitation center, familiar places within the community, or important places at the job site (e.g., restroom or staff lounge). These maps should be kept in the individual's memory notebook for reference at any time.

TRANSITIONAL LEARNING COMMUNITY
LEISURE ACTIVITY PLANNING SHEET

Name: _____ Date: _____

Leisure Goal: _____

ACTIVITY INFORMATION

Activity: _____ Activity Date: _____

Location Address & _____ Hours of Activity: _____
Telephone #: _____

Approximate Cost: _____

Independent _____ Semi–independent _____
Guests _____

MOBILITY PLAN

_____ Taxi _____ TA Van _____ Bike _____ Other
_____ Handivan _____ Bus _____ Walk

To Activity		Return		
Bus Number _____		Bus Number _____	Approximate Cost: _____
Time _____		Time _____	
Where _____		Where _____	
Transfer # _____		Transfer # _____	
Time _____		Time _____	
Where _____		Where _____	

Before Leaving, Check

Medication _____ Sign out/in _____
Notebook _____ Other _____
Money _____

Time	Time Management Plan

In Time Management Plan please include departure time, hours spending at activity and return time.

Total Cost of Activity $ _____

Case Manager _____ Date _____ Recreation Therapist _____ Date

TLC090492   LS009

Figure 5–3. Form used at the Transitional Learning Community for planning leisure activities.

Information Organizers

Individuals with memory or organization challenges may need assistance in creating systems for organizing and retrieving useful everyday information. One example is the use of an accordian file to store and retrieve information on community resources and personal papers (Milton, 1985). Condeluci et al. (1987) developed a form to help individuals track the receipt and payment of household bills, as shown in Figure 5–4.

Memory Notebook

Memory logs, journals, memory notebooks, or daily planners are all titles given to an external means of compensating for memory and executive

Month ___*May*___

Monthly Bill	Date Received	Date Due	Date Paid	Check No.	Mailed
Mortgage		5/10	5/7	952	✓
Car		5/12	5/9	955	✓
Orthodontist		5/4	5/1	942	✓
Cable TV	4/28	5/10	5/7	951	✓
Credit Union		5/15	5/10	964	✓
Department Store	5/1	5/25	5/19	973	✓
Electric	5/1	5/30	5/26	975	
Telephone	5/10	5/30	5/26	976	
Water	4/20	5/15	5/10	963	✓
Insurance (Car)	4/20	5/20	5/15	970	✓
School Loan		5/10	5/7	950	✓
Dr. Smith	5/3	5/15	5/10	962	✓
Gasoline	4/20	5/14	5/10	961	✓
Misc. Bills					
Air Cond. Repair					
Book Club	5/6	5/30	5/26	977	
Mag. Sub.					
Taxes					
Car Repair	5/17	5/17	5/17		NA

Figure 5–4. Illustration of a form used to organize and monitor bill paying. *Note:* From "Independent Living: Settins and Supports" (p. 330) by A. Condeluci, S. Cooperman, and B. Self, 1987. In M. Ylvisaker and E. M. Gobble (Eds.), *Community Re-Entry for Head Injured Adults*, Austin, TX: Pro-Ed. Copyright 1987 by Pro-Ed. Reprinted by permission.

functioning failures. This is a very commonly used strategy and has been found to be superior to use of mnemonic strategies (e.g., acronym formation) and repetitive drills (e.g., verbal or written rehearsal) in assuring that adults with brain injuries retain specific work-related information (Zencius, Wesolowski, & Burke, 1990).

The notebook should contain information that an individual will need on a daily basis, with the exact composition of the memory notebook highly individualized. For example, one individual had problems spontaneously recalling where different therapies were held within the facility and difficulty reading and using a simple map. Her cued spatial memory, however, was one of her strengths. Polaroid pictures were taken of the doors of each therapy office or group treatment area and paired with the name of the therapy session. She was then able to independently get herself to modules.

Possible sections to be included in a memory notebook, as suggested by Sohlberg and Mateer (1989c), include: *Orientation* for autobiographical information, *Memory Log* for recording hourly information regarding the activities of the individual, *Calendar* for recording appointments and future events, *To Do List, Transportation* for maps and bus information, *Feelings Log* for charting feelings in specific situations, *Names* for lists of therapists, family members, and so on, and *Today at Work* for recording information about work duties.

Giles and Clark-Wilson (1993) suggested two additional sections that may be useful for some individuals. A visitors section can be used to record accounts of visitations. These authors also recommended two prospective memory sections, one for *Things I Need To Ask* and a separate one for *Things To Remember To Do*. O'Hara and Harrell (1991) provide samples of notebook forms used in their program.

Although memory notebooks are valuable tools for compensating for memory deficits and are used on a frequent basis in rehabilitation settings, many adults with brain injuries fail to adequately use this technique or fail to use notebooks outside the rehabilitation setting. Sohlberg and Mateer (1989c) developed a three-stage process for training the use of memory notebooks. In the first stage, the Acquisition Stage, the individual must be able to state the name, purpose, and use of each of the notebook sections. In the second, or Application Stage, the individual learns and demonstrates the appropriate method for using the notebook through the role playing of situations. During the Adaptation Stage the individual is required to demonstrate the appropriate use of the notebook in structured functional settings, such as on a community outing.

Sohlberg and Mateer (1989c) offer several recommendations to assure functional use of any memory aid system: (a) The individual must keep the notebook with him or her at all times, both in therapy and in the community, (b) All staff and family members must be trained to understand and assist in the implementation of the notebook, (c) The therapist must ensure that the notebook reflects the functional needs of the individual, and (d) The therapist must understand that extended periods of training are often required for individuals with severe memory needs and should not prematurely discontinue training.

Electronic Devices

With the technological advances that have been made in the last decade, there are a variety of small, useful electronic devices, such as those listed in Table 5-1, that can be useful in specific situations for particular persons (Parenté & Anderson-Parenté, 1990; Parenté & DiCesare, 1991). Watches are a necessity, but care must be taken to select one that works for a client. Digital watches are generally easier for telling the time, but a model with the day and date of readable size on the same face as the time should be selected. One disadvantage is that digital watches often are not as simple to reset for time changes as traditional analogue watches.

Parenté and associates (Parenté & Anderson-Parenté, 1990; Parenté & DiCesare, 1991) identify a number of additional devices that can be used. Electronic credit-card-sized phone dialers or telephones with memories for storing and dialing numbers automatically can increase efficiency in placing calls. Data bank watches or personal information filers can be programmed (generally by some other person) with messages that will beep at a certain time to remind an individual of an appointment, an errand, or the need to take medication. Someone returning to school can conveniently use a microcassette recorder to record lectures for later

Table 5-1. Electronic devices for use as external aids.

Digital watch	Provide time, day of week, date
	Prompt actions with alarms
Electronic phone dialers, phones with memory	Store, dial frequently used phone numbers
Databank watches	Store messages, appointments
Microcassette recorders	Record lectures, directions, messages
	Store recorded messages for use on phone
Electronic pill boxes	Signal time to take medication
Personal beepers	Remind persons to take medication or action
Signaling devices	Sound for locating keys, wallet, car
Electronic spell checkers, dictionaries	Check spelling, definitions of words
Computers	Stimulation, management of information, generation of checklists, schedules

listening and taking notes. Recorders also can be used on the job to record instructions or to take phone messages. This permits individuals to replay the information for additional processing or to write down instructions at their own pace.

Electronic pill cases may be helpful in certain cases. The problem is having a sounding device within hearing distance at the correct time. Personal beepers can be used to remind individuals to take medications or perform activities. A number of devices will signal the location of an object such as keys, a wallet, or a car. Most are small sounding devices that emit an audible tone at the sound of a clap or whistle. Sound alarms for cars can be used to signal the location of a car in a parking lot. Electronic spell checkers or dictionaries also may be helpful for some individuals.

The most expensive electronic aid is a personal computer. Computers can generate checklists, store personal information, organize financial affairs, or assist with job or school responsibilies. Parenté and Anderson-Parenté (1990) describe the use of sophisticated operating system shells (such as user-friendly icons) to enable persons to use computers more easily at work. Schacter and Glisky (1986) propose the use of computers to train domain-specific knowledge. Software for checking spelling and grammar is helpful for many persons who must compose reports or letters.

The major obstacle in use of most electronic devices is their complexity. Multiple steps are generally involved and ongoing use requires the memory capacity to retain instructions. Another consideration is if the person will actually use the device. The individual may forget they even have the device (Moffat, 1984). A final consideration is whether the expense is justified, if a workable low-tech alternative strategy is available.

Environmental Adaptation

As stated in Chapter 4, environmental manipulations or modifications are changes made to an individual's social and physical environment that enable him or her to perform adequately despite significant impairments. Determination of appropriate modifications can be made by a clinician, after the evaluation and diagnostic therapy process, through careful observation of problems encountered by an individual in natural settings and a thorough understanding of the person's functional limitations.

Proposed environmental changes should be discussed with the individual to assure concurrence with the recommendations. In some instances, an individual may require training in the actual use of an adaptation. For example, if it is decided that an individual would benefit from a checklist placed on the door, as a reminder to get certain items before leaving in the morning, that individual may require cueing to refer to the checklist and reinforcement for using it until a habit is established. The advantage of most environmental adaptations, however, is that no change is required of the individual, rather increased independence and success are achieved through modification of the environment. As previously stated, the more severe the impairment in a particular cognitive-communicative process, generally the greater the required emphasis on environmental changes versus personal compensatory strategies.

Types of Environmental Adaptations

Environmental adaptations vary in scope and complexity. Some of the types of modifications, outlined by Szekeres, Ylvisaker, and Holland (1985), follow.

Physical Changes to the Environment

This category includes changes, such as removal of distracting items or noise from the environment, to facilitate processing and productivity or changing the location of objects in the environment to accommodate limitations. Examples of physical modifications within the living environment include the placement of orientation, memory, or planning devices or checklists in visible locations, weekly placement of medication in memory-jogging pill boxes to facilitate an accurate medication regimen, and labeling of kitchen cabinets and drawers. An example within a school setting would be placement of an individual near the front of the classroom and away from a window to limit distractions and to increase the teacher's ability to monitor attention and comprehension.

Some individuals make use of adaptations on their own. One individual known to the author placed a phone book in the middle of her kitchen floor as a reminder to tell her husband about a phone message when he came home from work. She could remember most phone messages, but would forget to tell him about the actual call. Her physical limitations made writing difficult and this technique worked for her.

Routines

Maintaining a set routine or structure often facilitates effective behavior after brain injury. The predictability and familiarity of established schedules or sequences of activities decrease the cognitive effort that is required. Especially when the individual has a severe memory problem or frontal lobe dysfunction, set routines, schedules, or patterns of interaction are an important management strategy.

Personnel

This strategy considers the value of persons around the individual to optimize performance. The use of a job coach to assist an individual in learning a job is an example of this adaptation. For individuals returning to school, consideration might be given to the teaching styles of various teachers to select the one that best matches the needs of the individual. A tutor may be employed to assist in a weak subject.

Communication Style

The communication style of persons in the environment can affect an individual's performance. Due to processing limitations, it important that staff and family reduce the rate, complexity, and amount of information provided to an individual and that they allow an individual maximum time to process and respond. Aggressive behavior or noncompliance often can be managed by careful examination of the communication style used with the individual and subsequent modification (Ylvisaker, Feeney, & Urbanczyk, 1993a, 1993b).

Establishing effective communication styles among staff, family members, individuals served, and other significant persons is a major consideration for successful rehabilitation. Ylvisaker et al. (1993a, 1993b) outline a framework and training program for developing a "positive communication culture." Five categories of communicative competencies are presented: content of communication, form of communication, encouragement of communication, environment for communication, and demonstration of respect in communication. Interactive training for all levels of staff and for family members is proposed, as well as coaching by a trained communicator in both simulated and natural situations. The goal of the training proposed by Ylvisaker, Feeney, and Urbanczyk (1993b) is to achieve better outcomes by developing positive and effective communication behavior among all persons involved in the rehabilitation process. The program they developed is an excellent method for incorporating family and residential staff into the rehabilitation process.

Expectations

This category includes the establishment of more realistic expectations for the individual or more appropriate requirements of performance. An example is reduction in the course load for a student or permitting an individual to take only a few courses when transitioning back to school. This compensates for the extra time that the person requires to read texts, prepare homework, and study for tests and enhances the likelihood of success in the courses taken. On the job, specific duties can be tailored to an individual's abilities or the time the person spends at work can be gradually increased to build up endurance.

Most rehabilitation programs are designed to provide maximum structure and environmental support at the beginning of the program and wean the individual to the level that is needed to retain effective performance over time. When adaptations are being proposed, the clinician should consider how intrusive the adaptation is and incorporate the particular individual's preferences. If the individual is in a residential program, the clinician must have a clear understanding of all the adaptations that have been made and communicate them to the family or other interested parties before the time of discharge, to promote the transfer and generalization of functional abilities to the discharge setting.

Rebuilding Language Abilities

Individuals with significant language deficits, such as anomia, reduced vocabulary comprehension, or poor spelling, may need retraining in these areas before attempting more functional-integrative tasks. Working on these specific language deficits may be critical to success in other areas of rehabilitation and to achievement of long-range vocational goals. Many methods of compensation for cognitive, behavioral, and executive deficits require at least a basic level of language skill. For example, individuals with memory problems need to record all appointments and upcoming events on a calendar. Individuals with initiation problems may need to use a checklist to keep moving from one activity to another. If an individual learns to express his or her feelings effectively, behavioral outbursts might be avoided.

Therefore, an early goal in treatment should be to address those communication skills needed for the individual to achieve treatment goals. The speech-language pathologist should work with other members of the treatment team to identify areas of need to ensure that an individual has the communicative abilities to benefit from each treatment area. Examples of how the speech-language pathologist can support the goals of other disciplines are given in Table 5-2.

As the communication expert on the rehabilitation team, the speech-language pathologist has the responsibility of assisting others in their communication with the individual. This includes educating others around the individual—the family, the rehabilitation staff, attendants, friends, and employers. They need to understand the nature of the cognitive-communication deficits and what areas are being targeted for improvement. Information can be provided on how to best communicate with the individual and what works best for the individual. This is particularly needed when an individual's communication patterns are different from what therapists may typically encounter. One way of disseminating such information is to write suggestions for communicating with an individual, such as in a memo as shown in Figure 5-5. This information could also be discussed in a team meeting. At other times, demonstration of the client's optimal performance may be helpful, so all members of the team understand what to reinforce from the individual. The speech-language pathologist should also provide information on how to redirect or cue an individual when performance is less than optimal.

Table 5-2. Examples of cognitive-communicative treatment tasks that support the work of other rehabilitation specialists.

Support of Occupational Therapy

Developing time concepts so individual can accomplish morning routine in a timely manner

Developing understanding of spatial and directional terms needed in mobility training

Training in the categorization of foods and household items in preparation for shopping (e.g., spaghetti would be on pasta aisle)

Developing a list of preferred foods from which menus can be generated

Training in sequencing of steps in common household routines, such as washing clothes, taking a shower

Building skills in reading of labels and directions on food packages

Building spelling skills of number words or use of a written list for accurate check writing

Support of Vocational Services

Developing alphabetizing skills when needed for a clerical job

Building reading skills for job related manuals

Developing specific speaking skills needed for a particular job, such as answering the phone or giving directions to preschool children

Developing the ability to understand directions and methods for self-determination of comprehension

Developing specific vocabulary needed on job, such as names of tools

Developing job interview skills

Developing the ability to respond to feedback from supervisor

Support of Therapeutic Recreation

Developing use of phone book and newspaper as sources of information

Developing use of phone to inquire about services, make arrangements

Building reading skills for planning worksheets

Helping learn how to read and order from a menu

Helping learn how to ask for directions to locations (e.g., restroom, bus stop)

Effective communication is necessary for efficient learning to occur within rehabilitation. The speech-pathologist should explore firsthand, through observations and probes within other treatment areas, if necessary, an individual's ability to process information in other therapies and the need to build compensatory strategies or suggest adaptations.

Example. David was one of those unusual persons who had a persisting fluent aphasia after a closed head injury. He engaged in casual conversation with minimal problems, was very personable and generally socially appropriate. His terrible temper come out at times, however, especially when he felt he or someone else was being treated unjustly. In addition, he was reported to be noncompliant by some therapists. After a few weeks into his program, David would become angry and leave during the middle of each of his vocational training sessions. When the speech-language pathologist

To: All Program Staff
From: Speech-Language Pathologist
RE: Communication Strategies for Sharon

Sharon has significant difficulty understanding instructions and group discussions. The problem is inconsistent because her world knowledge and her knowledge of word meanings is so patchy. In addition, she is rather "concrete" in her interpretations and she has difficulty making inferences. Therefore, she cannot make use of the context to determine what is meant nor can she see how the information is applicable to her life. Although she generally asks for clarification when she does not understand, there are times that she does not understand and is afraid to say so. She becomes angry and confused because she misinterprets what you say or doesn't know why you would say that. She also is not aware of how others perceive her in social situations and unwilling to change without understanding why.

Examples of problems that have occurred:
1. I said "Watch your facial expressions." She didn't know how she could "watch" her own face in the group situation. She could not interpret that phrase nor make use of the context to detect the meaning.
2. Working on her tone of voice and altering the level of politeness of requests, depending upon the social status of the listener: In talking about it and saying how we can alter politeness, she couldn't see how that was relevant because she felt she was always polite and would never speak harshly to someone regardless of their social status. Only after several real-life examples and videotaping of role play situations did she catch on.

Therefore, to communicate with her:
1. Keep your instructions straightforward and very explicit, with simple terms. Don't expect her to infer any steps unless she has gone over the task several times before.
2. Make sure she knows *why* she is being asked to do the task and why it has relevance to her life.
3. Avoid use of idiomatic expression, flowery terms, abstract terms or general phrases;
   Ex: Don't say: Give John a hand.
         Do say: Help John with his _____

         Don't say: You need to get on with your rehab.
         Do say: You need to focus on achieving your goals of _____
4. Watch her facial expression for signs she may not understand (frown, puzzled look) and ask her to say back what she is to do or the information you have said.
5. Give concrete examples of what you mean. In group discussions, if you start with a generalization, give several concrete examples and even think of an example that might be particularly relevant to her life.
   Example: It's important for a worker to get along with his/her supervisor.
   (Very general; she'd be uncertain how this is relevant to her)
   Give real-life examples:
   For instance, if your boss tells you to follow a set of instructions and you think you know an easier way of doing the task, what should you do? Do it your way, do it his way, or ask for permission to alter the instructions?
   Then give examples from her own life if possible:
   Sharon, remember when the occupational therapist became upset with you because you did not follow the directions on a package? You had made that dish many times before and knew an easier way to do it. What would have been a better way to handle this situation?
6. Avoid humor, jokes, teasing, at least at first. She is not able to understand what is meant or how it is meant to be taken (is person making fun of me?).

Figure 5-5. Example of a memo from the speech-language pathologist to other team members regarding communication strategies.

talked with David and the vocational counselor, the origin of the problem was immediately discovered. David had been assigned tasks, such as listening to an audio recording to follow directions and completing abstract, written directions. The speech-language pathologist listened to the tape and realized that the quality of the much used tape made it hard to understand. Combined with a significant auditory processing problem, this task was extremely frustrating, if not impossible, for David. In addition, the written directions were too complex for David's limited language abilities. The speech-language pathologist was able to work with David and the vocational couselor to identify tasks that would be better suited for David.

In all cases, care should be taken to select materials or content for language training that have functional relevance. For example, for an individual with limited language comprehension, vocabulary and comprehension training could focus on functional needs, such as understanding terms related to an individual's medications or understanding terms used on the treatment schedule. Almost all severely injured individuals will have some degree of difficulty in naming (Sarno, 1980, 1984b). Confrontation naming drills, however, have limited functional relevance, except to teach compensatory strategies. Consideration should be given to work on retrieval within more functional activities such as scripts for functional activities and discourse training. These are discussed later in this chapter.

Pharmacologic Management

As mentioned in Chapter 3, many individuals with brain injury may take medications for management of behaviors or ongoing medical conditions. In some instances, medications, such as some listed in Table 3–4, have been used to improve cognitive-communicative functioning. Psychostimulants, including Ritalin® and amphetamine, have been used to increase arousal and attention (Zasler, 1991). Catecholaminergic neurotransmitters, such as bromocriptine or Sinemet® (levodopa plus carbidopa), have been shown to improve physical, cognitive, and behavioral functioning after brain injury (Lal, Merbtiz, & Grip, 1988). Other medications, including some anticonvulsants (Dilantin® and phenobarbital), muscle relaxants (e.g., Valium®), and neuroleptics (e.g., haloperidol) may have an adverse effect on cognitive functioning (Zasler, 1991).

As stated previously, it is important that the clinician be aware of medications that an individual is taking and the potential side effects. Although many of the common medications and potential side effects were summarized in Table 3–4, the reader is encouraged to study the excellent reviews of pharmacological treatment after brain injury in Gualtieri (1988), O'Shanick and Parmelee (1989), O'Shanick and Zasler (1990), and Zasler

(1991, 1992). Of particular interest to speech-language pathologists is Zasler's (1992) brief review of studies on pharmacologic management of speech and language disorders.

Establishing Motivation for Communication Training

One of the first considerations in developing communicative competence is establishing the motivation for building effective social communication. As Spitzberg and colleagues (Spitzberg & Hurt, 1987; Spitzberg & Huwe, 1991) suggest, the desire to interact competently, to create a favorable impression, is a key factor in achieving communicative competence. Although often overlooked, building motivation is especially important for individuals who have sustained a brain injury. As mentioned several times, frontal lobe dysfunction can cause a lack of drive and difficulty in perceiving changes caused by the injury. Therefore, the individual may demonstrate reduced motivation for rehabilitation or appropriate social interaction.

Consideration first must be given to the level of the individual's awareness of deficits and readiness to change. Persons who are able to acknowledge their needs and express willingness to work on these areas have better treatment outcomes (Deaton, 1986; Lam et al., 1988). One suggestion for dealing with denial is to balance positive, or supportive, and negative (confrontational) feedback, emphasizing the desired behaviors rather than desired verbalizations (Deaton, 1986). Concrete feedback designed to focus an individual's attention on the consequences of deficits is important with individuals with brain injuries, because of abstract thinking limitations. Lam et al. (1988) provide the following examples of concrete feedback techniques: videotaping, use of computers, group therapy, situational assessment, family and peer feedback, planned failure, and supervised community outings.

Even without a brain injury, training in social communication can be tricky with adolescents or young adults for whom biases, social immaturity, or attitudes may interfere with full participation. Adolescent "rebellion" may make it difficult to discuss social norms and conflicts. Persons in this age range are trying to establish their identity and independence, but sometimes lack insight into ramifications of their behavior and the need to be socially responsible.

The clinician must employ a number of motivational techniques to obtain and keep the interest and motivation of individuals in treatment. Ben-Yishay and colleagues (1989) make use of peer and family pressure, metaphors, dramatic therapeutic activities, exhortation, and inspiration to induce committment to behavioral change. Ylvisaker and Holland (1985) suggest that the therapist be a coach who establishes a strong clinical relationship with an individual to increase motivation.

For individuals capable of learning from direct instruction, motivation can be heightened by establishing the importance of social relationships and of communication skills for effective social interaction, human growth and development, and maintenance of good mental health (Liberman et al., 1989; Riccardi & Kurtz, 1983). The clinician might begin by discussing the benefits of social relationships. As shown in Table 5–3, on a tangible level, good social relationships, whether with friends or family, help us obtain material needs or receive aid, such as when someone gives a present, does a favor, or lends a piece of equipment. Close relationships with others provide a sense of belonging or security. Affection, intimacy, companionship, and nurturance are additional benefits of interpersonal relationships. Social supports are vital resources for problem solving, reality testing, and coping with stress. Through successful social interactions, individuals achieve a better picture of their own identity and self-esteem.

Effective interpersonal communication is the key to meaningful social relationships (Liberman, 1982; Liberman et al., 1989). Communication is necessary for initiating and maintaining personal relationships, exchanging information, and expressing feelings. Through communication, people negotiate misunderstandings, direct the behavior of others, and learn the social rules of the community. Improved communication can lead to better interpersonal problem solving, increased coping, and improved self-confidence and self-esteem.

Skill in listening and speaking increases the options a person has in life. The choices of friendships, jobs, and living options all increase with improved communication. Many problems in life can be avoided through effective communication.

Table 5–3.   Benefits of social relationships.

Important material needs source

Assistance in achieving goals

Affection

Nurturance

Reliable alliance

Companionship

Reality testing

Modeling

Problem solving

Empathy and ventilation

Enhancement of self-worth

One point to make is that all persons have difficulty at times in being effective communicators. Few people are at ease when speaking in front of a group, as in advocating for construction of federal housing to the city council, or when attempting to settle a conflict with someone. There are techniques, however, that all persons use to help prepare for difficult situations (Liberman, King, DeRisi, & McCann, 1975). One way is by watching someone considered to be a skilled communicator and modeling that behavior. Another way is to ask a skilled friend for assistance in deciding what to say. A third way is through rehearsal and practice, either alone or with a friend.

Another point is that effective communication is, to a great extent, a learned, not innate, skill (Riccardi & Kurtz, 1983). Although we are born with a need and capacity for social interaction, our skill level is influenced by experience and training. Only through breaking communication into its component skills, learning about these skills, and actually practicing these skills do we become effective communicators.

Establishing and maintaining motivation for treatment of social communication must be an ongoing process. Active participation of an individual with TBI in goal setting is critical. An initial consideration is to help individuals identify their strengths and weaknesses. Aspects of their communication that are ineffective and aspects that are effective can be identified through joint viewing of a videotape by the clinician and the individual (Haarbauer-Krupa, Henry et al., 1985; Sohlberg & Mateer, 1989b). The results of the evaluation must be explained in functional language, not in professional jargon, with real-life examples being helpful for individuals to fully understand the areas to be addressed in treatment. As mentioned several times, techniques for self-monitoring always should be incorporated into treatment.

Addressing Affective Components

The effect of affective (emotional, personality) components on social communication were discussed in Chapter 2. Depression, high social anxiety, learned helplessness, and low self-esteem are often present after brain injury and contribute to poor interpersonal relationships and social isolation (Ellis, 1989; Newton & Johnson, 1985). It is important that these adjustment issues be dealt with in a holistic approach to brain injury rehabilitation by a psychologist well acquainted with the changes caused by brain injury.

Although the effectiveness of traditional psychotherapy with this population has been questioned, more appropriate models of psychotherapy have been developed (Ben-Yishay & Lakin, 1989; Prigatano, 1987; Prigatano et al., 1986). Ben-Yishay and colleagues developed a model for therapy aimed at assisting individuals in examining themselves, confronting their feelings and emotions, and establishing a new self-identity. The involvement of significant others in the rehabilitation process is an essential element of their approach. Significant others are encouraged to create an alliance with the therapist to induce behavioral change and a commitment to rehabilitation by the individual. Through the successes an individual achieves after these changes, improved attitude and greater life satisfaction are likely to occur (Ben-Yishay & Lakin, 1989).

Ben-Yishay and Lakin (1989), Prigatano (1989), and Haarbauer-Krupa, Moser et al. (1985) all emphasize the need to provide treatment within the context of a community. By creating a therapeutic "milieu," individuals can experience a sense of belonging, develop a support network, and learn to take responsibility for their actions. A community or "milieu" hour each day in which staff and the persons served come together provides an opportunity for clinicians to discuss emotional and behavioral issues in a therapeutic manner (Prigatano, 1989). By placing treatment within the context of a group or community setting, greater pressure exists for individual members to adopt and follow the group norms. The greater the cohesiveness of a group, the greater the pressure on individuals to conform to group norms (Sampson & Marthas, 1990). This helps to motivate individuals and to build greater acceptance of rehabilitation goals, leading to increased confidence and self-esteem. It also creates a supportive environment in which the individual can feel comfortable and accepted. Personal adjustment to disability can be facilitated through this mechanism.

Meichenbaum (1993) describes a number of techniques from the area of cognitive behavior modification (CBM) that have relevance to adjustment issues after brain injury. CBM, he states, includes various types of self-control training to improve self-efficacy and self-esteem. Collaboration between a client and significant others is emphasized, as well as interventions to help a client deal more effectively with emotional issues. Some of these techniques are described later in this chapter.

Rebuilding Stored Knowledge

In Chapter 2, the importance of stored knowledge on the processing and production of communication was discussed. After brain injury, an individual often demonstrates a reduction in stored knowledge or difficulty accessing stored knowledge. Problems are also frequently noted in the use of organizational strategies for storing and retrieving information. For example, individuals may have lost the ability to classify or associate concepts. This affects functional skills in many ways, including organizing a closet or work space or locating items within a certain section of a store.

Reduced understanding of everyday concepts is one aspect of impaired semantic memory that is frequently found after severe TBI. Attempts to build vocabulary through simple exercises, such as matching words to definitions, are not generally effective even for nondisabled individuals. New vocabulary is best learned through use in understandable contexts, such as within reading of a story or multiple sentences within appropriate situations. Therefore, concepts selected should be those that have functional significance to an individual, those that the individual needs for functioning as independently as possible in his or her environment (Valletutti & Dummett, 1992). A list of categories of functional vocabulary from Valletutti and Dummett is provided in Table 5–4.

A number of additional concepts become important when the concern is for social relationships (Gallagher, 1991; Valletutti & Dummett, 1992). One is reciprocity, or the idea that friends reciprocate in doing things for one another. For example, if someone invites you over for dinner, you reciprocate by inviting that person over for dinner next. Additional concepts important in building social knowledge include relationship concepts about friendship, empathy, other-orientation, supportiveness, trust, openness, and relationship building. Other concepts are intrapersonal, including self-identify, self-monitoring, self-discipline, and self-respect, with others being extrapersonal, such as society, convention, and conformity. Many social concepts have to do with regulation of interactions. These include cooperation, sharing, duties and responsibilities, fairness, manners, politeness, etiquette, morals, values, respect for others, cleanliness, and privacy.

As stated earlier, training in concepts is most effectively accomplished when it is conducted as part of a functional activity or in the context of a functional activity. For example, planning an airline trip to visit a family member can be the basis for developing concepts such as transportation, airports, clothing, weather, vehicles, fairness/conventions (waiting in lines), and responsibility (notifying family if plane will be late). Several clinicians have demonstrated the advantage of building word-finding or semantic abilities within a discourse format with children (Bedrosian, 1985; German, 1987). Techniques in this area are outlined in the next section.

Some individuals who have sustained a brain injury have an adequate store of knowledge, but have lost easy access because of disruption in semantic organization or inability to use effective strategies for storing and retrieving information (Hux et al., 1993; Gruen et al., 1990; Levin & Goldstein, 1986). Hux and colleagues (1993) recommend that treatment be aimed at improving semantic structure and integration. Semantic mappings of narratives used on a repeated basis would have more functional significance than attempts to improve semantic organization in general, they state. If an individual is capable of using information concerning

Table 5–4.   Categories of functional concepts.

Parts of face and body
Bodily functions
Foods and beverages
Eating utensils
Cooking utensils and equipment
Household appliances
Rooms of the house
Household items, materials, and equipment
Household tasks
Household cleaning supplies and equipment
Articles of clothing
Washing and grooming materials and equipment
Furniture and furnishings
Vehicles
Pets and plants
Weather conditions
First aid materials
Relationship names (father, mother, uncle, etc.)
Stores and shops
Service people in community (e.g., doctor, mail carrier, etc.)
Sports and sporting events
Recreation sites (movies, bowling alleys, parks, etc.)
Hobbies, arts, crafts, games
Careers and occupations
Salary, minimum wage, employee, employer, benefits
Net and gross pay, deductions, taxes, contributions
Community agencies and centers (library, hospital, post office, etc.)
Community businesses and industries
Restaurants and prepared foods
Dating and sex-related terms
Community activities
Legal matters, including civic duties
Travel and transportation
Household service personnel (electricians, plumbers, etc.)
Rent, leases, down payments
Financial transactions
Social Security
Hospitalization and insurance
Ecology, pollution, recycling, conservation
Diversity, race, nationality, religion, ethnicity, disability

Note: From *Cognitive Development: A Functional Approach* (pp. 42–45) by P. J. Valletutti and L. Dummett, 1992, San Diego: Singular Publishing Group. Copyright 1992 by Singular Publishing Group. Reprinted by permission.

semantic organization strategies, he or she should be trained in this. Pehrsson and Denner (1988) demonstrate the use of semantic organizers (also called semantic maps or webs), particularly for use in reading and writing tasks.

Szekeres and colleagues (Haarbauer-Krupa, Moser et al., 1985; Szekeres, 1992; Ylvisaker, Szekeres, Henry, Sullivan, & Wheeler, 1987) present methods for improving the organization of semantic memory and training in the use of organizational strategies. The use of visual aids often facilitates recognition of patterns or guides the organization of information. Haarbauer-Krupa, Moser et al. (1985) make use of a feature analysis chart to guide retrieval of information regarding a concept. This written guide cues the individual to think of associated items, the superordinate category, the function of the item, its physical properties, and its usual location.

Funtional organizational activities include organizing clothes within a person's bedroom closet and dresser, outlining aisles and departments of a local grocery store and classifying food items, and discusssing types of stores or departments within a large store and where to go to purchase different items.

Intervention often is necessary, as well, to assist individuals in seeing the organization of social situations and recognizing that there are patterns in how language is used in social situations. This increases their awareness of the expectations of others about communicative behavior. These different organizational schemata, described in more detail in Chapter 2, include:

1. Communication is based on the principles of reality and cooperation.
2. Conversation must adhere to Grice's maxims of quantity, quality, relevance, manner, and ambiguity.
3. Conversation is organized through turn taking.
4. Communication must be adapted to the audience.
5. Communication must be adapted to the setting and purpose.
6. There are scripts for common situations or communication goals.
7. There are schemata for various types of discourse.

A visual representation of the conversational rules may be a helpful treatment tool. This provides a written form of the guidelines to consider in all social interactions. One such representation is shown in Figure 5–6. This diagram is available in poster form from Thinking Publications. (See Appendix M, Functional Cognitive-Communication Material Sources.) It highlights Grice's maxims, as well as the importance of taking turns, mutual cooperation, and appropriate listening skills.

The second set of rules has to do with adaptation of communication to a physical and social context. One rule covers consideration of the degree of intimacy between the communication partners. People generally select topics and vary the degree of self-disclosure based on the closeness of the

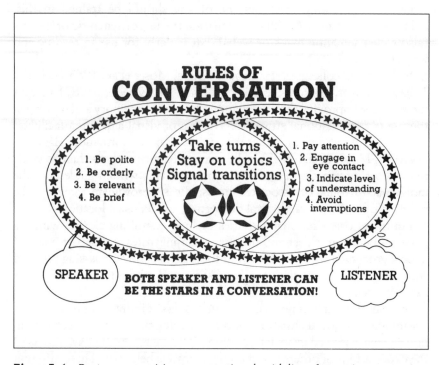

Figure 5-6. Poster summarizing conversational guidelines for use in communication training. *Note*: From *Daily Communication* (p. 123), by L. Schwartz and N. L. McKinley, 1984, Eau Claire, WI: Thinking Publications. Copyright 1984 by Thinking Publications. Reprinted by permission.

relationship. For example, introduction of topics such as sexual preferences, personal finances, and personal health conditions are appropriate with a spouse or boyfriend/girlfriend, but not with someone on the bus, an acquaintance, or even most friends.

One way to teach this is through use of drawing a circle such as the one in Figure 5-7 and contrasting topics that would be appropriate for each level. Safety issues to be highlighted include talking to acquaintances about personal issues or financial resources or being overly friendly with strangers. For example, Tami did not see anything wrong with discussing her medical problems or private life with cab drivers and apparently discussed many personal issues with one particular one. She was taken aback when he asked her out.

Other issues that can be discussed at this time include ensuring that one has the attention of another person and judging the degree of interest before starting a conversation. This is particularly important when approaching less familiar persons. A final consideration is how long to engage in conversation with a person at each level.

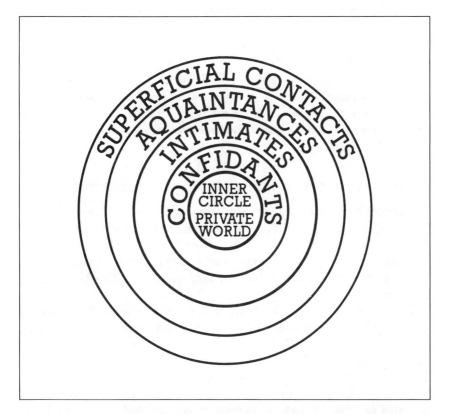

Figure 5-7. Structure for differentiating levels of intimacy and appropriate levels of self-disclosure. *Note:* From *Daily Communication* (p. 13), by L. Schwartz and N. L. McKinley, 1984, Eau Claire, WI: Thinking Publications. Copyright 1984 by Thinking Publications. Reprinted by permission.

Other communication schemata include a life script of the individual, scripts for everyday activities, and discourse structures (Szekeres, 1992). To help an individual organize information about his or her past and to provide an "algorithm" for telling others about his or her life, a form can be used to help the individual list significant life events.

The scripts of everyday life events, such as the one given in Table 2-5, can be role-played with the individual. It is particularly helpful to role-play events right before the individual must actually perform the script in real life, for example, role-playing going to the doctor the morning before an individual has an appointment. This provides the opportunity to outline behavior expected of the individual in such a situation and to practice language (e.g., stating symptoms of illness or concerns clearly and concisely) needed in a situation (e.g., a medical appointment). Social skills training is one method for teaching social "scripts" and are covered later in this chapter.

Rebuilding Functional Communication Skills

All the strategies discussed to this point are important in rebuilding functional communication skills. This section addresses a variety of specific methods for rebuilding discourse abilities in both individual and group treatment formats. First, are methods specifically addressing comprehension, then production of discourse is covered. Next, dyadic or small group activities addressing both areas are explored.

Comprehension and Retention of Spoken Information

The importance of good listening skills was highlighted in Chapter 3. Many people do not listen well "even though it is the primary requirement for effective communication" (Riccardi & Kurtz, 1983, p. 102). Processing of both interpersonal-oriented language as well as message- or idea-oriented language should be trained, because the two may differ (Horowitz & Samuels, 1987).

The first step might be to identify both verbal and nonverbal behaviors that individuals believe a good listener should demonstrate. These include:

1. Looking at the other person,
2. Showing interest by nodding, smiling,
3. Acknowledging comprehension and reinforcing the speaker through verbal expressions such as "mmm," "yes," "really,"
4. Asking questions on the topic,
5. Asking for clarifications of what is said, if needed,
6. Adding feelings and thoughts on the topic,
7. Summarizing what has been said.

General strategies for improving listening in interpersonal situations are suggested by Riccardi and Kurtz (1983) and Schwartz and McKinley (1984). These ideas include:

1. Prepare to listen, both mentally and physically, by discontinuing other activities or thoughts.
2. Shift completely from the speaker to listener role. Focus your attention on the speaker, not what you will say next.
3. Use active thinking in the listening process by mentally repeating key ideas or associating what is said with previous related knowledge.
4. Do not interrupt until the speaker has finished, even to ask for clarification.
5. Control judgmental responses or emotional evaluations.
6. Allow the speaker sufficient time to speak before taking a turn.

Training in the comprehension and retention of paragraph-length spoken material is a task that has much in common with everyday needs. The purpose is to increase the individual's ability to comprehend and state the main ideas and supporting details in information heard. Pre- and posttreatment testing can be conducted through use of the *Discourse Comprehension Test* by Brookshire and Nicholas (1993), in which the stimuli are narratives, or use of the expository paragraphs in Freeman, Mittenberg, Dicowden, and Bat-Ami (1992). Strategies for increasing performance in this area, including those from Freeman et al. (1992) and Haarbauer-Krupa, Henry et al. (1985), are listed in Table 5–5.

One method for improving listening is to build the ability to identify the *wh-* information from messages or other units of information. The individual can use the "Sun" diagram found in Haarbauer-Krupa, Henry et al. (1985) and Szekeres (1992) to record the information. A simplified form for *wh-* recording information is shown in Figure 5–8 and may be helpful in training individuals in selection of key information from messages or other spoken information. Other functional listening tasks include requiring the individual to listen to a message and determine whether there is information that is irrelevant or missing (Schwartz & McKinley, 1984).

The ability to follow spoken directions is a skill needed by all workers, as discussed in Chapter 3. Many workbooks include exercises that involve the following of progressively longer and more complex spoken directions for performing actions. Other exercises involve following of directions involving spatial concepts and maps (Schwartz & McKinlay, 1984). The use of strategies, such as those listed in Table 5–5, should be incorporated into the training procedures.

Table 5–5. Strategies for improving comprehension and retention of spoken paragraphs.

1. Notetaking of key concepts in memory notebook.
2. Training in self-monitoring of comprehension (cueing to "stop and think") and asking for repetition or clarification as needed.
3. Verifying that the information was understood by restating it in own words.
4. Training the individual to use visual imagery (translate words into "video" in head) to facilitate retention and recall.
5. Feedback from staff on use of strategies, reinforcement.
6. Use of subvocal rehearsal and elaboration of information.
7. Audiotaping of information for additional repetitions at a later point.
8. Training individual to recognize factors that interfere with comprehension (e.g., rate, amount, duration, competing stiumlation, complexity) and to request the needed adjustments directly to speaker.
9. Training in detection and use of organizational patterns of information to recall key information (e.g., who, what, when, where, why; main ideas and supporting details).

Get the Facts!

Who:	
What:	
When:	
Where:	
Why:	
How:	

Figure 5-8. Illustration of a structured format for isolating important information.

Training in listening is particularly important for individuals who plan to be in an academic environment. Listening in school settings requires among the most specialized listening skills; a more intense, active process of attention, greater selectivity in information gathering, and greater monitoring of comprehension are necessary for comprehension in an academic environment (Horowitz & Samuels, 1987). In contrast to listening in social situations, listening in school settings involves processing of propositions and arguments, analysis, and synthesis.

Training is needed in understanding the relationships between ideas and in detecting the main ideas and supporting details of what is heard in a lecture. Most lectures, newscasts, or speeches are planned and organized in some manner. Listeners can often profit from training at perceiving the speaker's schema or organizational structure (Devine, 1982).

According to Horowitz and Samuels (1987), most academic material is expository discourse, characterized by the discourse structures of: *attribution* (list-structure), *adversative* (comparison and contrast), *covariance* (cause and effect), and *problem—solution*. Devine (1982) provides two additional organizational patterns, *time sequence* in which events are provided in chronological order, such as in biographies, narratives, or science directions, and *generalization plus example* with a general statement followed by examples supporting the statement. Detection of these organizational structures which are listed in Table 5-6 can be facilitated by recognizing the cohesive ties, or signal words, that indicate transitions and key points within a discourse. Examples of these words are shown in Table 5-6, as well.

To a great extent, reading and auditory comprehension parallel one another (Horowitz & Samuels, 1987). Therefore, activities can be presented through either modality when working on higher level comprehension skills.

Discourse Production

Targeting Patterns of Discourse

One technique for building functional communication abilities is through discourse production tasks aimed at building the organization, informativeness, fluency, and cohesion of linguistic output. The purpose of discourse tasks would be to improve underlying language and nonlinguistic cognitive deficits within a functional skill (i.e., discourse) and to target specific aspects of discourse production noted as abnormal in the evaluation process.

Table 5-6. Discourse organizational patterns and examples of words that signal the organizational structure.

Organizational Patterns	Signal Words
Time Sequence Narration, Directions, Chronology	First, second, third; today, tomorrow; next, then, finally; in the past; soon
Simple Enumeration Attributes, Lists, Descriptions, Categories	In addition, also, furthermore, moreover, The four types are
Generalization plus Example	The most important, for example, for instance, thus
Covariance Cause and effect	As a result, so, accordingly, therefore, if-then
Adversative Comparison and contrast	However, but, on the other hand, in contrast
Problem-solution	In response, because, for these reasons

Treatment in this area should be based on an individual's profile of discourse production. Hartley and Jensen (1992) note that individuals who have experienced TBI often fit one of three profiles of discourse production: confused, impoverished, and inefficient discourse. An example of each is shown in Table 5–7.

Confused Discourse. In the first profile, individuals produce "confused" discourse, characterized by a high amount of inaccurate information and use of unclear phrases and nonindexed pronouns. Although they speak at a near normal rate of speech, much of what they say consists of dysfluencies, such as repetitions or revisions. These individuals also demonstrate significant language and memory impairments on standardized tests. Appropriate intervention for these individuals includes activities

Table 5–7. Examples of the three discourse profiles identified by Hartley and Jensen (1992).

Confused Discourse
[This woman thi-] this old man is walking down the street/ and when he doesn't notice it there's [a] a bulldog next to [him] him/ and well he knows there's a bulldog next to him/ and then he walks/ and then [he] he gets hit in the head by a pot/ and [he] he cusses at the lady/ and then he goes up to her house and come to find out it's an old lady/

Impoverished Discourse
A man was walking down the street/ and a dog bit him/ he kissed the lady's hand/

Inefficient Discourse
It looks like perhaps [um] this man owns [a] a little dog/ and they were walking here by a building [or] or [a] into a building/ which I can't really tell exactly [by] by the picture or the size of the picture, but perhaps into a building/ [uh] when [uh] something kinda plopped on the top of his head/ apparently somebody's little flower was either tossed down towards him, or just simply somehow fell right about when the man was underneath and hit the man on the head/ the man turned around and apparently yelled upwards to where [the little f] the little, either the people or whatever was up there [y well]/ and at that same time his little dog kinda did the same/ he kinda ruffed a little bit and looked up and went, "woof woof woof"/ so they had enough of that, in any case, and went ahead and went on in the building/ and apparently they were going up/ and [uh] he knocked on this door with the little puppy still next to him/ and this lady opened up the door and had a bone [uh] to kinda give the puppy/ [uh] and the little dog got the bone and sorta [de] decided to just run on away now that he had what he wanted/ and [uh] at that time [the] the man just thought it was very nice for the lady to do that/ so he held her hand and gave her a kiss on the hand holding his hat up, that he was wearing/ [uh] and in the picture with his hat up like that [you can tell you know] you can just kinda see the little bump he had from the [uh] little flower set up that fell on top his head/

Note: [   ] indicates a maze; / indicates end of communication unit, or utterance.

to promote accurate interpretation of pictures and effective retrieval of nouns or noun phrases in discourse. Simple sequence cards, pictures of everyday activities, or retelling of brief stories can be used. In addition, the individuals can benefit from training in volitional use of pause time and slower speech to allow time for planning and to decrease impulsive responses before thoughts are organized. To get them to focus on the critical content, they may benefit from structured guides of what information to give, such as the one in Figure 5–8.

Impoverished Discourse. A second profile identified by Hartley and Jensen (1992) is labeled "impoverished" discourse, because these individuals demonstrate such marked reduction in both productivity and content of discourse. An example of this profile is given in Table 5–7. Individuals fitting this profile generate few words, use very short utterances, and speak very slowly. Dysfluencies are limited, but silent pauses are common. Greatly reduced content is characteristic and the content that is produced is very concrete and fragmented, lacking in an understanding of relationships and integration of ideas. These individuals use very few cohesive ties to link their utterances into a unified story.

Treatment for someone with this profile is aimed at increasing the amount of language produced. One way is through the provision of an external structure as a cue for increased output. If a person has difficulty listing all the steps to complete a task, sequence cards can be used. The individual is asked to put the cards in order and then give a sentence for each picture. Next, the pictures are removed, and the individual is asked to repeat the sequence of activities without the visual prompts.

Another strategy for increasing productivity is to provide an list of the important information (e.g., *who, what, when, where, how, why*) that the person is expected to include in a describing a picture or in summarizing information heard (Milton & Wertz, 1986). Another method for structuring output is to require the person to speak an increasing number of utterances to describe an object or picture. Individuals can be encouraged to elaborate on key elements and expand their output by relating their feelings and experiences about a topic.

These individuals also benefit from activities aimed at understanding cause-and-effect relationships, making inferences, detecting motivations, and personal relationships in narratives, so that ideas are tied together in a logical and more abstract manner. Norman Rockwell paintings can be used to have the individual infer the motivations and relationships of persons depicted. The use of cohesive ties can be facilitated through exercises aimed at use of appropriate conjunctions to relate utterances and use of pronouns only after clear referents have been provided.

Individuals with the impoverished discourse profile generally show limited initiation of social interaction and limited initiation of topics in conversation. Treatment can target the development of a greater variety of social skills in conversation. A checklist such as the one in Appendix L can be used to record competency and use of each social skill and to sequence intervention so an increasingly greater variety of skills is employed.

Bedrosian (1985) identifies specific treatment strategies for increasing the conversational behaviors in individuals with low initiation. These include increasing the use of greetings and farewells, expressing needs, requesting information, and requesting repair. Specific ways to increase topic maintenance include use of acknowledgment and use of a general question such as, "What else can you tell me about this?" to maintain the conversation.

Inefficient Discourse. The third profile of discourse production from Hartley and Jensen (1992), as shown in Table 5–7, "inefficient" discourse, is characterized by use of accurate content, no inaccurate content, cohesive ties in the same frequency as noninjured speakers, and a normal rate of speaking. The difference is that these individuals speak longer, produce more words and utterances, and experience more dysfluencies than control speakers in the study. These are the speakers who provide excessive details, frequently revise what they say, and make tangential remarks.

The purpose of discourse tasks with these speakers is to increase the efficiency in conveying content. They benefit from explicit feedback about the quantity of verbal output and level of detail expected. Feedback should be provided regarding their excessive use of filled pauses or revisions and repetitions, along with training in self-monitoring of these behaviors (Whitney & Goldstein, 1989). Also needed are strategies to plan what to say and to stay focused on the purpose of a discourse. One strategy is to encourage reflective pausing for planning before speaking, perhaps providing the strategy with a catchy label, such as STP (stop, think, plan), as suggested by Ylvisaker et al. (1987).

Bedrosian (1985) suggests that treatment with a person with excessive verbalization should emphasize the turn-taking nature of conversation, plus listening and decreasing interruptions. A time limit can be set for each turn in a conversation (e.g., 20 seconds) or for the number of turns a person has per conversation.

Guidelines for organizing discourse are helpful for individuals with each of these profiles. Knowledge of the structural elements of discourse helps individuals see patterns to discourse that aid in the comprehension and generation of discourse. As listed in Table 5–6, both narrative and procedural discourse generally use a chronological time sequence. Procedural discourse involves telling someone how to do something or giving the directions to a particular location. Narratives include telling someone of a past event, such as an incident at work or an interesting experience, and telling of future plans. One strategy that most persons use when telling how to do something is to visualize a time when they have actually done the procedure and then tell each step as it is recreated in their mind (Graesser,

1978). Cohesive ties that mark transitions, or steps, such as *first of all, second, next,* and *finally,* should be encouraged to facilitate organization and sequencing.

There are several hypothesized structures of narratives or stories. Most researchers agree that narrative discourse requires that the speaker start with a setting followed by a series of actions given in an order primarily based on time. More specifically defined steps (Cannito et al., 1988; Stein & Glenn, 1979; Ulatowska et al., 1990) are:

1. Setting—The main characters are introduced, and the time and location of the story are given.
2. Initiating event—Something that happens leading the character(s) to think about trying to achieve some goal.
3. Internal response—The character has thoughts or feelings about the situation.
4. Attempt—The character takes action to reach the goal.
5. Consequence—This is the outcome of the character's actions, whether successful or not.
6. Reaction—The character's feelings or thoughts about the course of action or goal are reported.
7. Coda—A statement that indicates the end of the story.

Comic strips, videotapes, sequence cards, or complex pictures all can be used when teaching narrative structure. More unstructured tasks include having an individual tell what they did during a weekend or about a recently seen movie or TV program.

Small Group Discourse Tasks

A small group format is an excellent way to target functional communication skills. Some activities that can be used in small group or individual format to develop discourse processing and production are:

1. **Name That Person (or Object).** Slips of paper with names of objects or famous persons are made. In turn, each group member selects a slip, then provides clues for the other members to guess the name of the person or object.
2. **Get the Point.** A topic sentence is given to a person. The person is instructed to generate several sentences that will convey the main idea without actually repeating the exact statement (Schwartz & McKinley, 1984). The others try to guess the original main idea.
3. **Giving and Taking Directions.** A simplified map of a local area is passed to each member of the group. The person who will give directions is told to mark his or her house on the map. Then that person gives directions to the listener(s) for getting from a certain location (e.g.,

a mall, the bus station, the post office) to his or her house. The listeners are informed that they are to ask questions, if needed. At the end of the instructions, the listener(s) mark where they ended up and comparisons are made with the speaker's marked location. Listeners provide feedback to the speaker about the quality of the directions, what was helpful, and what, if anything was confusing.

4. **Stating Opinions on Topics.** Individuals are instructed to take a side on an issue, such as smoking in public areas, give an opinion, and then provide at least two supporting statements. This can be done in a dyad, with one person taking one side and the other taking the opposite side. This exercise is helpful to get individuals to maintain a consistent point of view on a topic, to think of ideas to substantiate an opinion, to think of ideas that will directly refute another's remarks, to be able to discuss a topic from varying perspectives, and to be able to disagree with someone without demonstrating anger.

Developing Conversational Skills

Treatment leading to effective interpersonal communication invariably involves the use of groups. General considerations on group treatment are in Chapter 4. Riccardi and Kurtz (1983) summarize the critical conditions for group treatment of interpersonal communication:

1. Isolation, definition, and presentation of essential skills or behaviors to be learned.
2. Practice of the targeted skills in simulated situations.
3. Provision for immediate feedback, including self-assessment and feedback from others.
4. Repetition and ongoing assessment of the targeted skill.
5. Provision of individualized goals within small group format.
6. Use of small group process to provide the support and stimulation for social learning.

Giving and receiving feedback is a crucial aspect of social skills training. Observational guides that outline both process and content skills can help structure the areas to be considered in giving feedback. It is generally necessary to provide ground rules for giving constructive feedback to other members of a group. A list of suggestions is given in Table 5–8. A primary concern is that, to be helpful, the feedback should be specific and descriptive without being judgmental (Riccardi & Kurtz, 1983). Labels and generalizations or inferences should not be used, only descriptions of the current behavior. Positive as well as negative feedback should be given, as in the sandwich technique. Alternatives or ways to improve performance can be given, but should not be provided as absolute answers.

Table 5-8.   Suggestions for giving constructive feedback.

Be descriptive, not judgmental.

Focus on the behavior, not the person.

Provide observations not inferences.

Speak for yourself.

Provide alternatives rather than answers.

Give feedback regarding behavior that works well as well as behavior that is not working.

Note: Based on material from Riccardi and Kurtz (1983) and Liberman, DeRisi, and Mueser (1989).

Being able to receive constructive feedback is not easy either. The receiver may need coaching to relax, breathe deeply, and listen carefully. The individual should be encouraged to ask for clarification, if needed, and to acknowledge valid points.

Modules Based on Pragmatics Model

There are many different ways of dividing the content for social communication training. Ehrlich and Sipes (1985) describe the content and format of a communication skills group they formed. A modular format was employed, with each module addressing specific behaviors within a general area of communication functioning. Four content areas were identified:

1. **Nonverbal communication**—paralinguistic features, facial expression, posture, eye gaze, and gestures;
2. **Communication in context**—topic initiation and maintenance, turn taking, and awareness of social context;
3. **Message repair**—awareness of communication breakdown, consideration of listener needs, and repair strategies;
4. **Cohesiveness of narrative**—sequencing of information, plus comprehension and use of spatial and temporal concepts.

Ehrlich and Sipes (1985) state that each session began with a definition and explanation of the skills to be learned. The therapists then modeled both inappropriate and appropriate examples of the target behavior. A videotape of these interactions was then reviewed for analysis and discussion.

The next step was for two individuals with brain injury to be videotaped while role-playing an assigned situation. Again the tape was replayed and group members were encouraged to provide feedback on the targeted behaviors, as well as specific behaviors that might have contributed to effective or ineffective communication interaction. At the end, the group members discussed the relevance of the module's theme to their own daily lives.

Ehrlich and Sipes (1985) developed a rating scale that they used to evaluate the performance of individuals in the group and determine progress in the group. This Communication Performance Scale is in Figure 3–2. A simplied version can be used for individuals to rate themselves after viewing the videotape of their role playing situation.

Ben-Yishay's Verbal Algorithms

Ben-Yishay and his staff at the Head Trauma Program of the New York University Medical Center developed a series of group exercises aimed at improving interpersonal communication (Ben-Yishay & Lakin, 1989; Ben-Yishay et al., 1980). One part of a multifaceted, holistic program, these exercises were designed as verbal "algorithms" useful in social situations and vehicles for working on cognitive, emotional, and acceptance issues. The group process was chosen to create a sense of social support and identity and to exert peer pressure for therapeutic benefit. The exercises were designed to help the members learn to express themselves clearly, read the feelings and thoughts of others, and develop a sense of self-worth.

The following specific exercise hierarchy was developed:

1. Introduce yourself.
2. Tell about two of your accomplishments (before injury).
3. Tell about two personal qualities you admire in yourself.
4. Tell another group member about qualities you admire in him or her.
5. Pretend you are a staff member and are interviewing a person who has applied to the rehabilitation program.
6. Evaluate your progress and any remaining problems in collaboration with a staff member.
7. Tell about qualities you respect in yourself.

Ben-Yishay describes the format of the group exercises as beginning with modeling by a staff member to demonstrate the desired performance. A group member then rehearses the exercise with additional staff modeling, if needed. After the individual completes the exercise, feedback is solicited from each group member in a "round robin."

Group Communication Activities

Sohlberg and Mateer (1989b, 1990) described several group activities they have found beneficial for addressing specific components of communication. One is titled the Hat Communication Activity and employs paper hats with directions, such as "Ignore me," "Interrupt me," "Compliment me," or "Ask me questions about myself," written on them. The hats are placed on each person's head without reading the messages. Then members of the group engage in conversation and respond to each other in the manner indicated on each person's head. At the end, participants try to guess what their hat said and discuss how they felt about the way others responded to them.

Another activity is the Party Activity where participants are given hypothetical identities to role-play in a party situation. Key aspects in this activity are introducing themselves and others and initiating conversation.

A third activity, Verbal Drawing Task, is a type of barrier game. One person must give instructions to another person to reproduce a particular drawing, involving three different shapes and two colors. At the end, the two drawings are compared to determine if and at what point communication broke down.

The fourth activity has each individual give an extemporaneous speech, at least 2 minutes long, to the group on a selected topic. The audience offers feedback on strengths and weaknesses.

Social Skills Training

Social skills training programs have a long history of use with a number of different clinical populations. Goldstein et al. (1980) offer the most detailed curriculum. Liberman et al. (1989) provide many helpful guidelines and additional social skills relevant to adult relationship situations, as well as forms for tracking progress. Burke (1988) and Johnson and Newton (1987) identify sets of social skills felt to be particularly relevant for most individuals with brain injury.

Social skills training offers a structured, systematic approach to rebuilding social communication. As demonstrated in Table 5-9, each communicative intent is taught in a script format. Goldstein et al. (1980) offer a hierarchy of skills, beginning with simple acts, such "Introducing Yourself," progressing to more difficult ones, such as "Answering a Complaint." More process-oriented skills, including setting a goal and gathering information, are also included in the Goldstein et al. (1980) curriculum.

Liberman et al. (1989) provide a more process and problem-solving approach to social skills training. They provide detailed examples of training people in "receiving," "processing," and "sending" skills. Common adult daily living and interpersonal interactions are identified, especially in the areas of friendship and dating. Also, they provide guidance for observing and tracking progress in social skills.

Wiig (1982a) developed a program for training communicative intents, or social skills, suggested for use with persons ages 9 to 21. The program includes decks of cards to provide practice for a certain communicative intent, such as asking a favor, or for communication within a functional

Table 5–9. Social skills training script for introducing yourself.

1. Choose the right time and place to introduce yourself.
2. Greet the other person and tell your name.
3. Ask the other person his/her name if you need to.
4. Tell or ask the other person something to help start your conversation.

Note: From *Skill-Streaming the Adolescent: A Structured Learning Approach to Teaching Prosocial Skills* (p. 91) by A. P. Goldstein, R. P. Sprafkin, N. J. Gershaw, and P. Klein, 1980, Champaign, IL: Research Press. Copyright 1980 by the authors. Reprinted by permission.

context, such as using the telephone. A simple map is included for training in giving directions.

Ylvisaker, Urbanczyk, and Feeney (1992) review literature on social skills training and offer ideas for combining behavioral and problem-solving/metacognitive approaches in teaching social skills to increase flexibility in performance. They, like Liberman et al. (1989), include grooming as an important aspect of social communication.

Helfenstein and Wechsler (1982) report the use of practice, coaching, videotaped feedback, and peer feedback to improve social interaction among individuals with TBI. They found that significant gains can be made in social skills through this process.

Applied Behavior Analysis

Applied behavioral analysis or behavioral management techniques can be used to extinguish undesirable behavior or to increase desirable behavior. Behavioral analysis begins by developing an objective definition of the target behavior in specific terms; assessing the frequency, duration, and intensity of the behavior; determining the conditions under which it is most and least likely to occur; and determining the consequences of the occurrence of the behavior (Lewis & Bitter, 1991). Behavioral intervention consists of the following steps: obtaining a baseline measure of the behavior of interest, implementing a behavioral program and measuring change in the behavior over time, and maintaining and generalizing the behavior (Wood, 1987). Jacobs (1993) provides valuable guidance and concrete examples for applying behavioral analysis strategies to brain injury rehabilitation.

Several single-case studies have demonstrated the effectiveness of behavioral intervention in altering maladaptive communication behaviors after brain injury. Giles, Fussey, and Burgess (1988) demonstrated the effectiveness of behavioral techniques on the conversational skills of an adult male who was verbose, with extreme tangentiality. The patient was trained to give responses that were less than 90 seconds in length in progressively more difficult situations, first answering questions that required a one-word response, then answering questions that required a phrase as a response, and finally unstructured conversation. Appropriate responses were rewarded with attention, praise, and chocolate. Inappropriate responses were punished by Time Out On The Spot (TOOTS), in which the clinician looked away for 20 seconds before interacting with the person. TOOTS was also used by the residential staff. Positive results were obtained and the training was discontinued after 1 month, with maintenance of appropriate responses at 2 months.

Another study by Lewis, Nelson, Nelson, and Reusink (1988) studied the effects of three types of feedback following inappropriate social communication. The participant was a 21-year-old male who had suffered a cardiac arrest and resulting anoxia. He exhibited impulsive and disinhibited social interactions. The number of socially appropriate and inappropriate comments was tallied for baseline and under three feedback conditions—attention and interest, ignoring, and correction. In the attention and interest phase, the therapist maintained eye contact, smiled, and showed interest in the participant. In the ignoring condition, the therapist broke eye contact for 3 seconds and then initiated a conversation on an appropriate topic. In the correction contingency phase, the therapist would tell the participant that he was talking nonsense and that he needed to start over and say something that made sense. The greatest decrease in socially inappropriate talking occurred in the correction contingency condition. Systematic ignoring was slightly less effective and, as might be expected, attention and interest greatly increased the problem. These researchers concluded that consistent correction of inappropriate behavior was an effective means of treating ineffective behavior. They emphasize the need for consistent responses from all staff and others in contact with an individual in order to alter behavior patterns.

One point that should be remembered is that while it is important to decrease or extinguish inappropriate communication behavior, at the same time, treatment should be directed to teaching and reinforcing appropriate behaviors that can replace maladaptive ones (Blackerby & Gualtieri, 1991). Many times, the challenging behavior is actually the way the person is communicating and more appropriate ways to have his or her needs met may need to be coached.

For example, one individual who had a very severe injury had difficulty remembering information. He often stopped people in the hall and asked them where he was supposed to be or where the next module was. All of this information was in his memory notebook. His redundant questions were decreased by a process of first saying, "Where can you find that information yourself?" and then later ignoring his questions. At the same time, he was taught other ways of initiating conversations. He was a very sociable person, and the clinician believed that one factor in his use of inappropriate questioning was his desire to interact with others. More appropriate strategies for initiating conversation provided a more success-ful substitute for the maladaptive behavior.

Development of Skilled Social Performance

Coping and Stress Management

To maintain effective cognitive-communication skills as functional de-mands increase, training in coping and stress management should be considered (Ponsford, 1990). Coping has been defined as "an individual's cognitive and behavioural efforts to master demands and conflicts" (Moore, Stambrook, & Peters, 1989, p. 171). Taylor (1983), in her model of cognitive adaptation in response to a life-threatening event, states that persons grapple with three major issues: (a) searching for a meaning in their experience, (b) attempting to gain mastery over the particular event and their life, and (c) making efforts to again feel good about themselves and restore self-esteem.

Studies indicate that avoidance strategies are often used for coping by persons with brain injury (Hinkeldey & Corrigan, 1990). For example, individuals with TBI were likely to use strategies such as "took it out on other people when I felt angry or depressed"; "refused to believe that it happened"; and "tried to reduce tension by smoking more." Moore et al. (1989) suggest that denial might be a coping mechanism used by some individuals to adjust to the long-term consequences of brain injuries. Professionals, they argue, should encourage feelings of control and a sense of well-being, even if this is not totally based in reality.

Ponsford (1990) suggests that rehabilitation should attempt to enhance coping after TBI by increasing the use of logical analysis strategies (e.g., considering several alternatives for handling a problem, trying to step back from a situation and be more objective) and information-seeking strategies (e.g., trying to find out more about the situation, talking with a profession-al person, and seeking help from persons with similar experiences).

Books on stress management (Charlesworth & Nathan, 1984; Quick & Quick, 1984) generally include three categories of strategies (Arokiasamy, Robertson, & Guice, 1993):

1. Strategies for preparing a person to deal with stress,
2. Strategies for organizing one's activities to reduce the impact of stress in one's life,
3. Strategies for dealing with particular stressful situations.

Preparing Oneself

This category includes ways of maintaining sufficient health for coping with life situations. Important stategies include exercising regularly, eating nutritional meals, practicing relaxation or meditation, and engaging in meaningful leisure activities. Activities that reduce coping abilities, such as using drugs or alcohol, working long hours, or negative thinking patterns, should be addressed. A comprehensive, holistic rehabilitation program should incorporate training in these areas. Hart and Hayden (1986) suggest coping training in progressive muscle relaxation and in heightening an individual's awareness of internal signs of tension.

Developing Habits that Mitigate Stress

This category includes general ways to reduce stress in life. Arokiasamy et al. (1993) include strategies such as using appropriate time management and avoiding procrastination, developing realistic expectations of what one can do within a certain period of time, minimizing confrontations with people and interruptions with activities, and prioritizing tasks. Another important strategy is development and use of a social support network.

Developing Strategies for Particular Situations

Two types of strategies in this category are direct stress reduction actions, or attempts to alter the source of stress, and palliative actions, attempts to self-regulate emotions resulting from a stressful experience. Direct means for dealing with a stressful situation include:

1. Leaving the situation,
2. Seeking additional data about the source of stress,
3. Breaking down a resolution plan into a smaller, more manageable plan of action,
4. Seeking outside help and/or advice,
5. Giving oneself time to adjust emotions, as in counting to 10.

Indirect methods include recognizing that there are limits to one's control over the situation, looking for humor in the situation, and re-framing one's view of the situation in a more positive outlook, as a challenge, or as a more positive experience. Hart and Hayden (1986) suggest developing a "script" or brief phrases that can be used by an individual to prepare for stressful situations or to deal with a problem. Positive self-statements, such as "I can do it" or "I can handle this," can be formulated and practiced to help a person cope in stressful situations.

A person's interests and preinjury coping style should be used in developing a coping strategy. One individual tended to become hostile to residential staff when he thought of previous situations that made him angry. He was a former computer programmer who maintained interest and skills with computers. It was found that working at his computer for even brief periods helped reduce his anger. Another individual tended to become angry at therapists giving him negative feedback. Having lived on a ranch all his life, he enjoyed the outdoors. With his therapists, he developed the strategy of working in the greenhouse on the grounds briefly between treatment sessions to "calm down."

Problem-Solving and Decision-Making Training

Training in problem solving and decision making is helpful for preparing individuals to in deal with difficult life situations. Ylvisaker et al. (1987) offer suggestions for working on this area. Most problem-solving training involves providing an individual with a structure that facilitates a step-by-step approach to problem solving, such as the guide shown in Figure 5–9 from Condeluci et al. (1987).

Following brain injury, some individuals have difficulty making daily life decisions, often because of disorganized thinking. Assisting individuals to develop a rational, reflective, and systematic method for making everyday decisions is of great functional significance (Valletutti & Dummett, 1992; Ylvisaker et al., 1987). A form that can be used to guide decision making is in Figure 5–10. Another example is provided by Ylvisaker and colleagues, who also suggest discussing the obstacles to effective decision making: impulsiveness, decreased judgment and safety awareness, misperception of a situation, cognitive distortions, inflexibility, and vulnerability to fatigue or attentional problems. Additional resources include Goldstein and Levin (1987), Schwartz and McKinley (1984), Sohlberg and Mateer (1989b), and resources listed in Appendix M.

Assertiveness Training

Assertion or assertiveness training was developed by Bandura (1969) to help persons overcome problems in expressing positive and negative feelings. Through observation and imitation of a model, persons are trained to communicate in an honest, self-assertive manner rather than a passive or aggressive manner. This type of training may be of benefit to individuals who are less cognitively impaired, particularly when they find it difficult to stand up for themselves or are having difficulty expressing feelings without excessive anger.

Assertiveness training begins by analyzing verbal and nonverbal characteristics of passive, assertive, and aggressive behaviors (Alberti & Emmons, 1982; Giles & Clark-Wilson, 1993; Holland & Ward, 1990). Role plays, observations, videotaped feedback, and peer discussion are used to contrast behaviors from each of these categories and to build and reinforce assertive behaviors.

Problem–Solving Sequence

1. What's the problem?

↓

2. What's your goal?

↓

3. What information do you need?

↓

4. Possible Solutions	Effective?	Acceptable?	Time?	Able?
a.				
b.				
c.				
d.				

↓

5. Which is the best solution?

↓

6. Make a plan of action.

↓

7. Carry out your plan

↓

8. Did it work? Why?

Figure 5-9. Illustration of a form used to facilitate problem solving. *Note:* From "Independent Living: Settings and Supports" (p. 331) by A. Condeluci, S. Cooperman, and B. Seif, 1987. In M. Ylvisaker and E. M. Gobble (Eds.), *Community Re-Entry for Head Injured Adults*, Austin, TX: Pro-Ed. Copyright 1987 by Pro-Ed. Reprinted by permission.

Developing Emotional Intimacy Skills

Blackerby and Gualtieri (1991) suggest several techniques for developing better social relationships or emotional intimacy. The first step is to teach the recognition and labeling of feelings and relating feelings with particular behaviors and outcomes. Learning how to express feelings or beliefs to

1. What am I expected to do? _____
   _____

2. Do I have all the information? _____

   What is the purpose? _____

   What is the cost in money? _____

   What are time requirements and constraints? _____

   What are required materials or equipment? _____

3. What are my alternatives and consequences? _____

Alternatives	Consequences
1.	
2.	
3.	
4.	
5.	

4. Do I need additional help or information? _____

5. Do I have abilities and requisities? _____

6. What is my plan? _____
   _____

7. How did it turn out? _____
   _____

Figure 5-10. Illustration of a form for facilitating a reflective decision-making process.

another person in a way that is clear and will not lead to resistance or resentment by the partner is an important step. Blackerby and Gualtieri (1991) suggest the use of "I" statements, generally also a part of assertiveness training, to express feelings. These are shown in Table 5–10. With this mechanism, the speaker accepts ownership for his or her feelings and, in the case of expressing negative feelings, suggests a way to compromise or resolve the situation.

The social relationship concepts discussed under Stored Knowledge are now discussed. Blackerby and Gualtieri (1991) suggest the use of some of the techniques developed as sensitivity training in the 1960s and 1970s to enhance the capabilities of individuals with brain injury to develop

Table 5-10. Guide for constructive feedback in interpersonal situations.

Expressing Negative Feelings or Feedback

I feel _____	Tell how behavior affects you
when you _____ ,	Describe other person's behavior
because I _____ .	Tell why you are affected that way
I would like _____ ,	Describe change you want
because _____ .	Tell why change important to you
What do you think?	Listen to other person's response.
	Be ready to compromise.

Expressing Positive Feelings or Feedback

I feel _____	Express positive emotion
when you _____ .	Identify the positive behavior

emotional intimacy in relationships. They emphasize that family members should be included in training in this area for successful intervention and generalization.

Dealing With Challenging Behaviors

As stated in Chapter 1, one of the major challenges to clinicians is dealing with the challenging behaviors that may occur after brain injury. The most commonly reported categories of behavioral issues include verbal and physical aggression, impulsivity, anxiety/irritability, sexual disinhibition, egocentricity, noncompliance, and at-risk behaviors, such as elopement (Fisher, 1985; Peters, Gluck, & McCormick, 1992; Wood, 1988). In the early stages of rehabilitation, these issues generally are addressed through close supervision, use of restraints, and medication (Peters et al., 1992). Individuals with some of these behaviors often are excluded from post-acute programs but other behaviors are common in this setting. Peters, Gluck, and McCormick (1992) suggest behavioral management techniques have been used successfully with some behaviorally challenged individuals in a community re-entry setting.

Noncompliance is a common problem faced in community re-entry programs and it is a major problem because it substantially interferes with an individual's ability to benefit from rehabilitation. Noncompliant behaviors include refusal to participate in therapy, failure to follow rules, failure to follow instructions, and inability to accept criticism and feedback (Zencius, Lane, & Wesolowski, 1991). Many reasons can contribute to an individual's failure to comply with his or her rehabilitation program. Therefore, the first step in managing noncompliant behavior is to assess the reason for the noncompliance (Zencius et al., 1991). Age and cultural differences may result in an individual's lack of interest in proposed activities, such as an outing to a museum. If the clinical program is rigid and does not address an individual's concerns and needs, an individual rightly may not want to participate. Memory problems may prevent an individual from remembering what is to be done or what is expected of them.

Once these issues have been sorted out and the noncompliant behavior identified as a target for intervention and antecedents and consequences analyzed, intervention can begin. The two methods of intervention described by Zencius et al. (1991) include antecedent control and consequence management. Consequence management includes techniques such as individual point systems, level programs, and behavioral contracts. Antecedent control techniques involve changing or structuring the environment to elicit or facilitate the desired behavior. This is the type of intervention needed when the noncompliance is due to memory failures. Written checklists, cueing through pictures, maps, and verbal cues are techniques that can be used to enhance compliance (Zencius et al., 1991).

Including the Family in Rehabilitation

One aspect of the disability movement has been the family support movement (Singer & Powers, 1993). Family systems theory also has had an impact, resulting in the recognition that major illnesses or chronic disabilities affect the whole family not just the patient. Treatment, therefore, should incorporate the family and assist the family in functioning as a unit. The family support movement gained momentum in the 1980s as parents and advocates for persons with disabilities urged policymakers to strengthen and empower families who are primary caregivers to persons with chronic disabilities.

It is not only appropriate rehabilitation philosophy to include the family, but a major requirement for rehabilitation facilities under standards of the Commission for the Accreditation of Rehabilitation Facilities (CARF). Unfortunately, there is uncertainty about how much family involvement is appropriate (Shaw & McMahon, 1990). Several writers have discussed the sources of conflict that may arise between a rehabilitation team and a family (McLaughlin & Carey, 1993; McNeny & Wilcox, 1991; Shaw & McMahon, 1990).

Family involvement is particularly critical at the postacute stage, when the goal is to return an individual to active social and community participation. The need to work with the family in identifying discharge goals was discussed in Chapters 3 and 4. It is important to identify specific needs and expectations of the family, as well. Kreutzer and colleagues have developed a Family Needs Assessment (Kreutzer, Camplair, & Waaland, 1988) to determine the family's needs (Kreutzer & Wehman, 1990). These needs generally change at the postacute stage, as the family comes to grips with the long-term consequences of an injury. By understanding family needs and expectations, staff can provide the appropriate education and support to facilitate the understanding necessary for setting and achieving realistic goals. A team cannot hope to obtain generalization of skills unless the family has been included in the rehabilitation process. Williams (1993a, 1993b) and Solomon and Scherzer (1991) offer considerations for developing better team-family interactions, ensuring positive family involvement, and providing appropriate supports for the family.

As Williams (1993a, 1993b) points out, clinicians should support families and individuals by identifying opportunities for choices, family participation, and resources available in the community. The family must be included in discussions on the rationale and importance of compensatory strategies. Williams also exhorts professionals to balance hope with realism and to introduce the families to both formal (e.g., local head injury support group) and informal (e.g., other families coping with brain injury) support systems.

DePompei, Zarski, and Hall (1988) emphasize how crucial it is to involve the family in training of communicative competence after brain injury. One of the major goals of cognitive-communication treatment should be "to maintain functional communication within the family" (p. 14). The family can assist in the recovery of communication abilities by supporting and reinforcing positive communication interactions. DePompei and co-workers (1988) provide strategies for decreasing family dysfunctional responses to an individual's cognitive-communicative deficits.

Working as Part of a Team

Being able to work as part of a team is an essential skill for any professional in brain injury rehabilitation, especially when the desired product is to achieve functional outcomes within efficient time frames. With the complexities of issues following brain injury, interdisciplinary collaboration and cooperation is a must, because no one professional or discipline is likely to singly accomplish the desired outcome. Each team member is expected to contribute in unique but overlapping ways to reach the desired end results. Wright and DeGenaro (1981) state that "an effective team is a cohesive, mutually supportive, and trusting group that has high expectations for task accomplishment but at the same time respects individual differences in values, personalities, skills, and idiosyncratic behavior" (p. 260).

As pointed out by Likert (1967), teams produce two types of products—the end product and the process product. In the case of rehabilitation teams, the end product is the achievement of effective and efficient outcomes for a client. To produce this product, each member must have a clear understanding of the mission and objectives of the rehabilitation program and the specific outcome goals for each individual served. Each team member is expected to contribute toward the accomplishment of the goals and objectives as identified by the entire team. This means each team member must demonstrate maturity and personal responsibility. Clarity and honesty in communication about responsibilities and expectations is essential. Team members must be accountable and dependable for assigned roles in achieving the end product. This includes completing documentation within designated time frames, being punctual to team meetings, and following through with assigned responsibililties.

Team process products include improved relationships, communication, decision making, problem solving, and conflict management (Wright & DeGenaro, 1981). Improvement in the team process facilitates but does not guarantee improvement in the end product (Wright & DeGenaro, 1981). Effective interpersonal communication and commitment to the group decision-making process are particularly critical skills for each member of an effective team (Likert, 1961; Ylvisaker et al., 1993b; Wright & DeGenaro, 1981). Team members must provide specific information, express their opinions clearly and succinctly, actively listen to and acknowledge the opinions and findings of others, and invite discussion and elaboration of ideas. Members do not interrupt or distract from others and they seek to keep interactions positive and supportive. Mutual trust and respect are displayed.

In the team process, each member is encouraged to provide input, with the understanding that creative or differing options can be expressed without undue criticism. The final plan of action, however, is one that is reached through group problem solving, compromise, and negotiation, so that the plan can be supported by all members of the team. Commitment to achieving and supporting a team consensus ensures that conflicts are dealt with inside the team and that a consistent point of view is presented to an individual, family, and funding source.

Flexibility and creativity are additional desirable characteristics for team members. Willingness to assist other team members or to adjust one's goals or schedule to accommodate other team members builds team strength and a spirit of support and cooperation. The willingness to look at new possibilities or approaches, to see possibilities not drawbacks in the proposals of others, and to go the extra mile to do what it takes to effect the desired outcome for an individual is highly valued in a team model of rehabilitation.

Professional training programs, unfortunately, rarely prepare new clinicians for team membership. It is important for a new team member to be given time to observe and absorb the team culture and norms and to develop ease with the group process. In addition, each professional must develop an understanding of the knowledge base and expertise of each other clinical professional and an understanding of how his or her own skills can contribute to the functional outcome goals.

Integration of Skills Into Functional Settings

All the techniques suggested in this chapter have been selected with consideration of generalization and transfer of skills in mind. However, as treatment progresses, a greater percentage of time should be spent in integrating the achieved skills into real-life situations.

Co-Treatment

Groups that are co-led by representatives from more than one discipline are excellent means for integrating individual goals across disciplines and helping to generalize cognitive-communication gains. Examples of possible groups are social skills training groups co-led by a psychologist and speech-language pathologist, job communication groups led by a speech-language pathologist and vocational counselor, community life training led by an occupational therapist and speech-language pathologist, and back-to-school groups led by a speech-language pathologist and neuropsychologist.

O'Hara and Harrell (1991) identify issues to be covered in a back-to-school group, including time management, study skills, notetaking, and reading comprehension training. Additional resources are in Appendix M as well as in the Volume 6, Number 1 issue of the *Journal of Head Trauma Rehabilitation*, National Head Injury Foundation publications, DePompei and Blosser (1991), and Blosser and DePompei (1989).

Carlson and Buckwald (1993) describe a vocational communication group they developed. At the author's facility, a Job Communication Group was established to cover interviewing skills, interactions with supervisors, and interactions with co-workers. Resources include programs developed for personal and social adjustment training with individuals in a vocational program. Some of these are listed in Appendix M.

Community-Based Treatment

A way to circumvent problems in generalization and transfer is to provide treatment within an individual's own environments. This "rehab without walls" approach has gained momentum over the last several years because of decreased funding, the desire of individuals with brain injury to have home-based rather than institution-based treatment, and the greater understanding of the long-term obstacles to successful reintegration.

In this approach, one clinician generally becomes the sole service provider developing and implementing strategies and training protocols within an individual's home, work, and community environments (Milton, 1985; 1988). Community-based supports and resources are integrated into such a program, as well (Kneipp & Paul-Cohen, 1993). For example, an individual is assisted in identifying and accessing local community resources such as fitness clubs, civic organizations, or community college classes to continue to improve in socialization, communication, and thinking. Social supports such as friends, church groups, family members, and local head injury support groups are enlisted to assist an individual in achieving his or her goals. Opportunities for volunteer work are pursued to provide structure to a person's day and a sense of contribution to society, as well as an opportunity for social interaction, problem solving, and learning. Kneipp and Paul-Cohen (1993) provide specific ideas of how to provide community-based services and supports.

In *vivo* training of social skills is a technique addressing communicative skills in the midst of routine life activities. Both Ylvisaker et al. (1992) and Wong et al. (1993) offer support for this approach.

Generalization to Discharge Community

Unless generalization issues are specifically addressed, individuals with brain injury often fail to use skills they have acquired in their residential rehabilitation program once they return home, and may even experience a decline in their abilities after discharge. One way to promote generalization of skills to the discharge community is to provide meaningful and specific documentation regarding the environmental adaptations and self-initiated strategies known to enhance an individual's behavior. Durgin et al. (1991) describe the use of a Client Resource Book (CRB) to specify the types of support an individual needs for living and working in discharge settings. It serves as a postdischarge reference for anyone who might need to work with an individual, for example, an employer. The various areas to consider, suggested by Durgin et al. (1991), are in Table 5-11.

If an individual with TBI has been in a residential program, another strategy is to have a clinician return home with the individual after discharge. This way the individual can be assisted in setting up the compensatory strategies or making the adaptations that are needed. When the individual will be returning to employment, a vocational placement specialist is valuable in assisting in the smooth transition to the work site.

Obstacles to a Functional Approach

Adopting a functional approach, especially working on social communication, has a number of obstacles, as listed in Table 5-12. The major problem is lack of training relevant for postacute rehabilitation. Therapists generally

Table 5–11. Content for Client Resource Book.

Skill Area	Content Examples
Cognition/Communication	Journal pages and strategies Communication goals and guidelines Memory strategies and aids Decision-making and problem-solving checklists Structured thinking or task analysis forms
Psychosocial	Personal coping strategies Special behavioral program or contract "I" statements
Daily Living Skills	Housekeeping schedule Menu planning sheets Budgeting forms Mobility planning sheets To Do Lists Shopping lists
Physical	Personal fitness plan Use and care of adaptive equipment Transfer or ambulation guidelines
Medical	Medication guidelines and monitoring forms Dietary recommendations Specific long-term medical needs Seizure log forms Referral sources in home community
Vocational	Resume/references Vocational strengths and limitations Task-specific vocational strategies Suggestions for supervisors Completed job application
Recreation	List of personal interests and options Community resources Leisure outing planning forms Community outing guidelines

Note: From "Programming for Skill Maintenance and Generalization" (p. 367) by C. J. Durgin, L. P. Cullity, and P. M. Devine, 1991. In B. T. McMahon and L. R. Shaw (Eds.), *Work Worth Doing: Advances in Brain Injury Rehabilitation*. Winter Park, FL: PMD Press. Copyright 1991 by PMD Press, Inc. Adapted by permission.

do not receive training that prepares them to build functional skills, to deal with social communication, or to handle difficult interpersonal behaviors. Because professional training in postacute brain injury rehabilitation or functional communication is limited, clinicians have to be flexible enough to change their conceptions of service delivery to assume a more functional approach. Those who have worked in acute medical settings may be

Table 5-12.   Problems faced in addressing functional communication.

Lack of training in functional skill development and social aspects of
  communication

Biases toward service delivery

Tendency to ignore or cover up embarrassing behavior because of own social
  learning

Lack of training in dealing with difficult behaviors

Inappropriate social behavior seen as a nuisance and not a target for treatment

Overestimation of real-life abilities

Failure to understand organic basis of behavior

Need for creativity and individualization of methods

accustomed to formal settings and fixed roles. They may not recognize the
need for and value of this approach and question billing to train an
individual for something as "ordinary" as grocery shopping.

I can remember one of the first individuals I worked with in a more
functional mode. I went, armed with paper and pencil tasks, to work with
Andy, a 29-year-old woman who had sustained anoxic damage from
respiratory arrest during the cesarean birth of her second child. The client
had transportation problems that day, so I volunteered to go to her home.
It was a chance to observe her interacting with her child, then 14 months
old. Andy would walk behind the child, saying "No! No!" as the toddler
explored the living room and tried to pick up objects. I dropped the
workbooks and spent the hour teaching the woman how to play with her
child, to reinforce the child's language and social behavior, and to redirect
the child rather than saying "No" each time. At first, it seemed odd to bill
for playing with a child, but the improvement noted in this mother-child
relationship overcame the initial uncertainty.

As noted by Crosson (1987), treatment in interpersonal communication is very difficult for many therapists. The tendency, based on the therapists' own social learning, might be to ignore or cover up awkward or embarrassing behavior. Therapists have to unlearn this tendency in order to
address such issues with individuals.

Dealing with some of the challenging behaviors after brain injury is, in
fact, difficult for even experienced clinicians. Confronting individuals with
brain injury about their undesirable behaviors may result in anger, and the
clinician may hesitate to place a potential wedge in an already questionable
relationship by providing sensitive feedback (Prigatano, 1989). Clinicians
need to know how to provide negative feedback in a manner that will be
easier for the individual to take.

Another obstacle in effecting change in social behavior is the tendency, at times, for a team to see interpersonal behaviors as a nuisance rather than a target for change (Crosson, 1987). This is particularly true when a team lacks leadership in the area of behavioral management or when a team, for whatever reason, operates with a bias toward acceptance of a given behavior from that individual. An example is Brenda, who had been a very strong-willed and attractive person, financially supporting herself from high school graduation and at age 28 working as a very successful independent cotton broker in Houston. She had been married only a year when she was hit by a drunken driver. She had severe ataxia with significant intentional tremors and severe challenges of attention, memory, and impulse control. She would interrupt others, take out her notebook in the middle of conversations, and not pay attention to what others said. She spoke in a harsh vocal tone and gave direct commands to others. She often displayed anger when she was not able to do things. Many times, she was allowed to continue with inappropriate behavior, perhaps because many of the therapists identified with her or felt sorry for her. However, this behavior resulted in many problems for her husband and family when she returned home.

Another obstacle is that therapists may not understand the organic basis of many behaviors and interpret them as being willful (Crosson, 1987). Problems in initiation may be mistakenly attributed to lack of motivation. Therapists sometimes make the mistake of assigning homework or designing a home program without considering problems in planning and initiation. Assignments go uncompleted because the appropriate structure is not in place.

Clinicians who see individuals with brain injury strictly in structured clinical settings tend to overestimate their real-life abilities. Therefore, they fail to realize the need to address functional cognitive-communication skills or to work with an individual within functional settings.

Another obstacle may be a lack of flexibility in an institution for scheduling or making community outings. A clinician may have to use creativity to overcome this obstacle. Opportunities for more natural interactions within the facility, such as in the cafeteria, gift shop, or library, should explored, as well as volunteer job trials within the institution.

A final consideration is that a functional approach is not an easy approach; it requires individualization of treatment and creativity on the part of a clinician.

The newness of the field of postacute rehabilitation means that it is constantly changing. This can be both challenging and stressful. Professional burnout is an issue supervisors must frequently deal with. However, the newness of the field means that no one person has the complete answer for how to conduct postacute rehabilitation.

Although several outcome studies demonstrating the overall effectiveness of postacute rehabilitation have been published in the last few years, many more studies are needed to discern the most effective and efficient treatment approaches for this population. Clinicians are encouraged to participate in efficacy studies to critically assess their own treatment. The final judge of our success is the degree of community integration that is achieved and maintained and the quality of life attained for the individuals served.

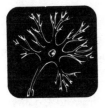

References

Adamovich, B. (1991). Cognition, language, attention, and information processing following closed head injury. In J. S. Kreutzer & P. H. Wehman (Eds.), *Cognitive rehabilitation for persons with traumatic brain injury: A functional approach* (pp. 75–86). Baltimore: Paul H. Brookes Publishing.

Adamovich, B. B., Henderson, J. A., & Auerbach, S. (1985). *Cognitive rehabilitation of closed head injured patients.* San Diego: College-Hill Press.

Adams, C., & Bishop, D. V. M. (1989). Conversational characteristics of children with semantic-pragmatic disorder. I: Exchange structure, turntaking, repairs and cohesion. *British Journal of Disorders of Communication, 24,* 211–239.

Adams, J. H., Graham, D., & Gennarelli, T. A. (1985). Contemporary neuropathological considerations regarding brain damage in head injury. In D. Becker & J. Povlishock (Eds.), *Central nervous system trauma status report-1985* (pp. 65–77). Bethesda, MD: National Institutes of Health, NINCDS.

Adams, J. H., Graham, D., Murray, L. S., & Scott, G. (1982). Diffuse axonal injury due to non-missile head injury in humans: An analysis of 45 cases. *Annals of Neurology, 12,* 557–563.

Adams, J. H., Graham, D., Scott, G., Parker, L. S., & Doyle, D. (1980). Brain damage in fatal non-missile injury. *Journal of Clinical Pathology, 33,* 1132–1145.

Alberti, R. E., & Emmons, M. L. (1982). *Your perfect right: A guide to assertive living* (4th ed.). San Luis Obispo, CA: Impact Publishers.

Alexander, M. P., Benson, D. F., & Stuss, D. T. (1989). Frontal lobes and language. *Brain and Language, 37,* 656–691.

Alexandre, A., Colombo, F., Nertempi, P., & Benedetti, A. (1983). Cognitive outcomes and early indices of severity of head injury. *Journal of Neurosurgery, 59,* 751–761.

Allen, R., & Brown, K. (1976). *Developing communication competence in children.* Skokie, IL: National Textbook Company.

American Speech-Language-Hearing Association. (1991). Guidelines for speech-language pathologists serving persons with language, socio-communicative, and/or cognitive-communicative impairments. *Asha, 33*(Suppl. 5), 21–28.

Annegers, J. F., Grabow, J. D., Kurland, L. T., & Louis, E. R. (1980). The incidence, causes and secular trends of head trauma in Olmstead County, Minnesota. *Neurology, 30*, 912–919.

Applegate, J. L., & Leichty, G. B. (1984). Managing interpersonal relationships: Social cognitive and strategic determinants of competence. In R. N. Bostrom (Ed.), *Competence in communication: A multidisciplinary approach* (pp. 33–55). Beverly Hills: Sage.

Arkowitz, H. (1981). Assessment of social skills. In M. Hersen & A. S. Bellack (Eds.), *Behavioral assessment: A practical handbook* (2nd ed., pp. 296–327). New York: Pergamon Press.

Arokiasamy, C. V., Robertson, J. E., & Guice, S. E. (1993). Effective strategies for directing and managing change in the rehabilitation setting. In C. J. Durgin, N. D. Schmidt, & L. J. Fryer (Eds.), *Staff development and clinical intervention in brain injury rehabilitation* (pp. 335–367). Gaithersburg, MD: Aspen Publishers.

Ashington, J. W., Harris, P. L., & Olson, D. R. (Eds.). (1988). *Developing theories of mind.* Cambridge, England: Cambridge University Press.

Aten, J., Caligiuri, M., & Holland, A. (1982). The efficacy of functional communication therapy for chronic aphasic patients. *Journal of Speech and Hearing Disorders, 47*, 93–96.

Auerbach, S. H. (1986). Neuroanatomical correlates of attention and memory disorders in traumatic brain injury: An application of neurobehavioural subtypes. *Journal of Head Trauma Rehabilitation, 1*(3), 1–12.

Axelrod, D. (1986). *Head injury in New York state: A report to Governor Cuomo and the Legislature.* Albany: Office of Health Systems Management, Division of Health Care Standards and Surveillance.

Backlund, P., Brown, K., Gurry, J., & Jandt, F. (1982). Recommendations for assessing speaking and listening skills. *Communication Education, 31*, 9–17.

Baddeley, A., Harris, J., Sunderland, A., Watts, K. P., & Wilson, B. A. (1987). Closed head injury and memory. In H. S. Levin, J. Grafman, & H. Eisenberg (Eds.), *Neurobehavioral recovery from head injury* (pp. 295–317). New York: Oxford University Press.

Bandura, A. (1969). *Principles of behavior modification.* New York: Holt, Rinehart and Winston.

Barco, P. P., Crosson, B., Bolesta, M. M., Werts, D., & Stout, R. (1991). Training awareness and compensation in postacute head injury rehabilitation. In J. S. Kreutzer & P. Wehman (Eds.), *Cognitive rehabilitation for persons with traumatic brain injury: A functional approach* (pp. 129–146). Baltimore: Paul H. Brookes Publishing Co.

Barry, P., & Clark, D. (1992). Effects of intact versus non-intact families on adolescent head injury rehabilitation. *Brain Injury, 6*, 229–232.

Barth, J. T., Alves, W. M., Ryan, T. V., Macciocchi, S., Rimel, B., Jane, J., & Nelson, W. (1989). Mild head injury in sport: Neuropsychological sequelae and recovery of function. In H. S. Levin, H. M. Eisenberg, & A. L. Benton (Eds.), *Mild head injury* (pp. 257–275). New York: Oxford University Press.

Bateson, G. (1972). *Steps to an ecology of mind.* San Francisco: Chandler.

Baxter, R., Cohen, S. B., & Ylvisaker, M. (1985). Comprehensive cognitive assessment. In M. Ylvisaker (Ed.), *Head injury rehabilitation: Children and adolescents* (pp. 247–274). Austin, TX: Pro-Ed.

Bedrosian, J. L. (1985). An approach to developing conversational competence. In D. N. Ripich & F. M. Spinelli (Eds.), *School discourse problems* (pp. 231–255). San Diego: Singular Publishing Group.

Bedrosian, J. L. (1993). Making minds meet: Assessment of conversational topic in adults with mild to moderate mental retardation. *Topics in Language Disorders, 13*(3), 36–46.

Bellack, A. S. (1983). Recurrent problems in the behavioral assessment of social skill. *Behavior Research and Therapy, 21,* 29–41.

Benoit, P., & Follert, V. (1986). Appositions in plans and scripts: An application to initial interactions. In D. G. Ellis & W. A. Donohue (Eds.), *Contemporary issues in language and discourse processes* (pp. 239–256). Hillsdale, NJ: Lawrence Erlbaum.

Benton, A. L. (1974). *The Revised Visual Retention Test* (4th ed.). San Antonio: The Psychological Corporation.

Benton, A. L., & Hamsher, K. (1983). *Multilingual Aphasia Examination* (rev. ed.). Iowa City: AJA Associates.

Benton, A. L., Hamsher, K. deS., Varney, N. R., & Spreen, O. (1983). *Contributions to neuropsychological assessment: A clinical manual.* New York: Oxford University Press.

Ben-Yishay, Y., & Diller, L. (1983). Cognitive rehabilitation. In M. Rosenthal, E. R. Griffiths, M. R. Bond, & J. D. Miller (Eds.), *Rehabilitation of the head-injured adult* (pp 367–378). Philadelphia: F. A. Davis.

Ben-Yishay, Y., & Lakin, P. (1989). Structured group treatment for brain-injury survivors. In D. W. Ellis & A-L. Christensen (Eds.), *Neuropsychological treatment after brain injury* (pp. 271–296). Boston: Kluwer Academic Publishers.

Ben-Yishay, Y., Lakin, P., Ross, B., Rattok, J., Cohen, J., & Diller, L. (1980). Developing a core "curriculum" for group exercises designed for head trauma patients who are undergoing rehabilitation. In Y. Ben-Yishay (Ed.), *Working approaches to remediation of cognitive deficits in brain damaged persons* (Rehabilitation Monograph No. 61). New York: New York University Medical Center, Institute of Rehabilitation Medicine.

Ben-Yishay, Y., Piasetsky, E. B., & Rattok, J. (1987). A systematic method for ameliorating disorders in basic attention. In M. Meier, A. Benton, & L. Diller (Eds.), *Neuropsychological rehabilitation* (pp. 165–181). New York: The Guilford Press.

Ben-Yishay, Y., Rattock, J., & Diller, L. (1979). A clinical strategy for the systematic amelioration of attentional disturbances in severe head trauma patients. In Y. Ben-Yishay (Ed.), *Working approaches to remediation of cognitive deficits of brain damaged persons* (Rehabilitation Monograph No. 60) (pp. 1–27). New York: New York University Medical Center, Institute of Rehabilitation Medicine.

Ben-Yishay, Y., Silver, S., Piasetsky, E., & Rattok, J. (1987). Relationship between employability and vocational outcome after intensive holistic cognitive rehabilitation. *Journal of Head Trauma Rehabilitation, 2*(1), 35–49.

Berko-Gleason, J. B., Goodglass, H., Obler, L., Green, E., Hyde, M., & Weintraub, S. (1980). Narrative strategies of aphasic and normal-speaking subjects. *Journal of Speech and Hearing Research, 23,* 370–382.

Beukelman, D., Yorkston, K., & Lossing, C. (1984). Functional communication assessment of adults with neurogenic disorders. In A. Halpern & M. Fuhrer (Eds.), *Functional assessment in rehabilitation* (pp. 101–115). Baltimore: Paul H. Brookes Publishing Co.

Bickhard, M. (1987). The social nature of the functional nature of language. In M. Hickmann (Ed.), *Social and functional approaches to language and thought* (pp. 39–65). Orlando, FL: Academic Press.

Bishop, D. V. M., & Adams, C. (1989). Conversational characteristics of children with semantic–pragmatic disorder. II. What features lead to a judgment of inappropriacy? *British Journal of Disorders of Communication, 24,* 241–263.

Blackerby, W. F., & Gualtieri, T. (1991). Recent advances in neurobehavioral rehabilitation. *NeuroRehabilitation, 1*(3), 53–61.

Blosser, J. L., & DePompei, R. (1989). The head-injured student returns to school: Recognizing and treating deficits. *Topics in Language Disorders, 9*(2), 15–33.

Bohnen, N., Twijnstra, A., & Jolles, J. (1992). Post-traumatic and emotional symptoms in different subgroups of patients with mild head injury. *Brain Injury, 6,* 481–487.

Bower, G. H., Black, J. B., & Turner, J. T. (1979). Scripts in text comprehension and memory. *Cognitive Psychology, 11,* 177–200.

Boyce, N., & Larson, V. (1983). *Adolescents' communication development and disorders.* Eau Claire, WI: Thinking Publications.

Bracewell, R. J., Frederiksen, C. H., & Frederiksen, J. D. (1982). Cognitive processes in composing and comprehending discourse. *Educational Psychologist, 17*(3), 146–164.

Braun, C. M. J., Baribeau, J. M. C., Ethier, M., Daigneault, S., & Proulx, R. (1989). Processing of pragmatic and facial affective information by patients with closed head injuries. *Brain Injury, 3,* 5–17.

Braun, C. M. J., Lussier, F., Baribeau, J. M. C., & Ethier, M. (1989). Does severe traumatic closed head injury impair sense of humour? *Brain Injury, 3,* 345–354.

Braunling-McMorrow, D., Lloyd, K., & Fralish, K. (1986). Teaching social skills to head injured adults. *Journal of Rehabilitation, 52*(1), 39–44.

Brooks, D. N. (1975). Long and short term memory in head injured patients. *Cortex, 11,* 329–340.

Brooks, D. N., Campsie, L., Symington, C., Beattie, A., & McKinlay, W. (1986). The five year outcome of severe blunt head injury: A relative's view. *Journal of Neurology, Neurosurgery, and Psychiatry, 49,* 764–770.

Brooks, D. N., McKinlay, W., Symington, C., Beattie, A., & Campsie, L. (1987). Return to work within the first seven years of severe head injury. *Brain Injury, 1,* 5–19.

Brookshire, R. H., & Nicholas, L. E. (1993). *Discourse Comprehension Test.* Tucson, AZ: Communication Skill Builders.

Brown, L. (1982). *Communicating facts and ideas in business* (3rd ed.). Englewood Cliffs, NJ: Prentice–Hall.

Burgess, F. W., & Alderman, N. (1987). Rehabilitation of dyscontrol syndromes following frontal lobe damage: A cognitive neuropsychological approach. In R. L. Wood & I. Fussey (Eds.), Cognitive rehabilitation in perspective. New York: Taylor and Francis.

Burke, W. H. (1988). Head injury rehabilitation: Developing social skills. Houston: HDI Publishers.

Burns, M. S., Halper, A. S., & Mogil, S. (1985). Clinical management of right hemisphere dysfunction. Gaithersburg, MD: Aspen.

Buschke, H., & Fuld, P. A. (1974). Evaluating storage, retention and retrieval in disordered memory and learning. Neurology, 24, 1019–1025.

Butler, K. G. (1990). The future of language science: Impact on clinical practice. In C. M. Shewan (Ed.), The future of science and services seminar (ASHA Reports No. 20) (pp. 51–57). Rockville, MD: American Speech-Language-Hearing Association.

Camplair, P. S., Kreutzer, J. S., & Doherty K. R. (1990). Family outcome following adult traumatic brain injury: A critical review of the literature. In J. S. Kreutzer & P. Wehman (Eds.), Community integration following traumatic brain injury (pp. 207–223). Baltimore: Paul H. Brookes.

Cannito, M. P., Hayashi, M. M., & Ulatowska, H. K. (1988). Discourse in normal and pathologic aging: Background and assessment strategies. Seminars in Speech and Language, 9, 117–134.

Carlson H. B., & Buckwald, M. B. W. (1993). Vocational communication group treatment in an outpatient head injury facility. Brain Injury, 7, 183–187.

Carr, E. G., & Durand, V. M. (1985). The social-communicative basis of severe behavior problems in children. In S. Reiss & R. Bootzin (Eds.), Theoretical issues in behavior therapy (pp. 219–254). New York: Academic Press.

Cavallo, M. M., Kay, T., & Ezrachi, O. (1992). Problems and changes after traumatic brain injury: Differing perceptions within and between families. Brain Injury, 6, 327–336.

Charlesworth, E. A., & Nathan, R. G. (1984). Stress management: A comprehensive guide to wellness. New York: Atheneum.

Cicerone, K. D., & Giacino, J. T. (1992). Remediation of executive function deficits after traumatic brain injury. NeuroRehabilitation, 2(3), 12–22.

Cicerone, K. D., & Tupper, D. E. (1986). Cognitive assessment in the neuropsychological rehabilitation of head-injured adults. In B. P. Uzzell & Y. Gross (Eds.), Clinical neuropsychology of intervention (pp. 59–84). Boston: Martinus Nijhoff Publishing.

Cicerone, K. D., & Wood, J. C. (1987). Planning disorder after closed head injury: A case study. Archives of Physical Medicine and Rehabilitation, 68, 111–115.

Coelho, C. A., Liles, B. Z., & Duffy, R. J. (1991a). Analysis of conversational discourse in head injured adults. Journal of Head Trauma Rehabilitation, 6(2), 92–99.

Coelho, C. A., Liles, B. Z., & Duffy, R. J. (1991b). Discourse analyses with closed head injured adults: Evidence for differing patterns of deficits. Archives of Physical Medicine and Rehabilitation, 72, 465–468.

Coelho, C. A., Liles, B. Z., & Duffy, R. J. (1991c). The use of discourse analyses for the evaluation of higher level traumatically brain–injured adults. Brain Injury, 5, 381–392.

Cole, L. (1989). E pluribus pluribus: Multicultural imperatives for the 1990s and beyond. *Asha, 31*(8), 65–70.

Committee on Government Operations. (1992). *Fraud and abuse in the head injury rehabilitation industry (House Report No. 102–1059; Committee's 35th Report).* Washington, DC: U.S. Government Printing Office.

Condeluci, A. (1992). Brain injury rehabilitation: The need to bridge paradigms. *Brain Injury, 6,* 543–551.

Condeluci, A., Cooperman, S., & Seif, B. A. (1987). Independent living: Settings and supports. In M. Ylvisaker & E. M. R. Gobble (Eds.), *Community re-entry for head injured adults* (pp. 301–348). Austin, TX: Pro-Ed.

Condeluci, A., & Gretz-Lasky, S. (1987). Social role valorization: A model for community re-entry. *Journal of Head Trauma Rehabilitation, 2*(1), 49–56.

Conger, J. C., Moisan-Thomas, P. C., & Conger, A. J. (1989). Cross-situational generalizability of social competence: A multilevel analysis. *Behavioral Assessment, 11,* 411–431.

Cooley, R. E., & Roach, D. A. (1984). A conceptual framework. In R. N. Bostrom (Ed.), *Competence in communication: A multidisciplinary approach* (pp. 11–32). Beverly Hills: Sage.

Cooper, K. D., Tabaddor, K., Hauser, W. A., Schulman, K., Feiner, C., & Factor, P. R. (1983). The epidemiology of head injury in the Bronx. *Neuroepidemiology, 2,* 70–88.

Cope, D. N. (1990). The rehabilitation of traumatic brain injury. In F. J. Kottke & J. F. Lehmann (Eds.), *Krusen's handbook of physical medicine and rehabilitation* (4th ed., pp. 1217–1251). New York: W. B. Saunders.

Crago, M. B., & Cole, E. (1991). Using ethnography to bring children's communicative and cultural worlds into focus. In T. M. Gallagher (Ed.), *Pragmatics of language: Clinical practice issues* (pp. 99–128). San Diego: Singular Publishing Group.

Crosson, B. (1987). Treatment of interpersonal deficits for head-trauma patients in inpatient rehabilitation settings. *The Clinical Neuropsychologist, 1,* 335–352.

Crosson, B. C., Barco, P. P., Velozo, C. A., Bolesta, M. M., Werts, D., & Brobeck, T. (1989). Awareness and compensation in post-acute head injury rehabilitation. *Journal of Head Trauma Rehabilitation, 4*(3), 46–54.

Cullity, L. P., Jackson, J. D., & Shaw, L. R. (1991). Community skills training. In B. T. McMahon & L. R. Shaw (Eds.), *Work worth doing: Advances in brain injury rehabilitation* (pp. 307–327). Winter Park, FL: PMD Press, Inc.

Curran, J., & Monti, P. (1982). *Social skills training.* New York: Guilford Press.

Daigneault, S., Braun, C. M. J., & Whitaker, H. A. (1992). An empirical test of two opposing theoretical models of prefrontal function. *Brain and Cognition, 19,* 48–71.

Damico, J. S. (1991). Clinical discourse analysis: A functional approach to language assessment. In C. S. Simon (Ed.), *Communication skills and classroom success: Assessment and therapy methodologies for language and learning disabled students* (pp. 125–148). Eau Claire, WI: Thinking Publications.

Davis, G. A., & Wilcox, M. J. (1985). *Adult aphasia rehabilitation: Applied pragmatics.* San Diego: College-Hill Press.

Deaton, A. V. (1986). Denial in the aftermath of traumatic head injury: Its manifestations, measurement, and treatment. *Rehabilitation Psychology, 31*(4), 231–240.

Deaton, A. V. (1991). Group interventions for cognitive rehabilitation: Increasing the challenges. In J. S. Kreutzer & P. H. Wehman (Eds.), *Cognitive rehabilitation for persons with traumatic brain injury* (pp. 191-200). Baltimore: Paul H. Brookes Publishing Co.

Delany, R. C., Rosen, A. J., Mattson, R. H., & Novelly, R. A. (1980). Memory function in focal epilepsy: A comparison of non-surgical, unilateral temporal lobe and frontal lobe samples. *Cortex, 16,* 103-117.

D'Elia, L. F., & Boon, K. B. (1993). *Handbook of normative data for neuropsychological assessment.* New York: Oxford University Press.

Delis, D. C., Kramer, J., Kaplan, E., & Ober, B. A. (1986). *The California Verbal Learning Test.* San Antonio, TX: Psychological Corporation.

Dennis, M., & Lovett, M. W. (1990). Discourse ability in children after brain damage. In Y. Joanette & H. H. Brownell (Eds.), *Discourse ability and brain damage: Theoretical and empirical perspectives* (pp. 199-223). New York: Springer-Verlag.

DePompei, R., & Blosser, J. L. (1991). Functional cognitive-communicative impairments in children and adolescents: Assessment and intervention. In J. S. Kreutzer & P. H. Wehman (Eds.), *Cognitive rehabilitation for persons with traumatic brain injury* (pp. 215-236). Baltimore: Paul H. Brookes Publishing Co.

DePompei, R., Zarski, J. J., & Hall, D. E. (1988). Cognitive communication impairments: A family-focused viewpoint. *The Journal of Head Trauma Rehabilitation, 3*(2), 1-112.

Devine, T. G. (1982). *Listening skills schoolwide: Activities and programs.* Urbana, IL: National Council of Teachers of English.

DiSalvo, V. S., & Steer, J. (1980). *An identification of communication skills and problems found in organization related careers.* Paper presented at the meeting of the Speech Communication Association, New York.

Dunn, L. M., & Dunn, L. M. (1981). *Peabody Picture Vocabulary Test—Revised.* Circle Pines, MN: American Guidance Service.

Durgin, C. J., Cullity, L. P., & Devine, P. M. (1991). Programming for skill maintenance and generalization. In B. T. McMahon & L. R. Shaw (Eds.), *Work worth doing: Advances in brain injury rehabilitation* (pp. 349-371). Winter Park, FL: PMD Press.

Ehrlich, J. S. (1988). Selective characteristics of narrative discourse in head-injured and normal adults. *Journal of Communication Disorders, 21,* 1-9.

Ehrlich, J., & Barry, P. (1989). Rating communication behaviours in the head-injured adult. *Brain Injury, 3,* 193-198.

Ehrlich, J., & Sipes, A. (1985). Group treatment of communication skills for head trauma patients. *Cognitive Rehabilitation, 3,* 32-37.

Einstein, G. O., McDaniel, M. A., Bowers, C. A., & Stevens, D. T. (1984). Memory for prose: The influence of relational and proposition specific processing. *Journal of Experimental Psychology: Learning, Memory, and Cognition, 10*(1), 133-143.

Eisenberg, H. M., & Weiner, R. L. (1987). Input variables: How information from the acute injury can be used to characterize groups of patients for studies of outcome. In H. S. Levin, J. Grafman, & H. M. Eisenberg (Eds.), *Neurobehavioral recovery from head injury* (pp. 13-29). New York: Oxford University Press.

Ellis, D. W. (1989). Neuropsychotherapy. In D. W. Ellis & A. L. Christensen (Eds.), *Neuropsychological treatment after brain injury* (pp. 241–269). Boston: Kluwer Academic Publishers.

Engelmann, S. E., & Carnine, D. W. (1982). *Theory of instruction: Principles and applications.* New York: Irvington.

Eslinger, P. J., & Damasio, A. R. (1985). Severe disturbance of higher cognition after bilateral frontal lobe ablation: Patient EVR. *Neurology, 35,* 1731–1741.

Ewert, J., Levin, H. S., Watson, M. G., & Kalisky, Z. (1989). Procedural memory during post-traumatic amnesia in survivors of severe closed head injury: Implications for rehabilitation. *Archives of Neurology, 46,* 911–916.

Falvey, M. A. (1989). *Community-based curriculum: Instructional strategies for students with severe handicaps* (2nd ed.). Baltimore: Paul H. Brookes Publishing Co.

Farrell, A. D., Rabinowitz, J. A., Wallender, J. L., & Curran, J. P. (1985). An evaluation of two formats for the intermediate–level assessment of social skills. *Behavioral Assessment, 7,* 155–171.

Fife, D. (1987). Head injury with and without hospital admission: Comparisons of incidence and short–term disability. *American Journal of Public Health, 77*(7), 810–812.

Fife, D., Faich, G., Hollinshead, W., & Boynton, W. (1986). Incidence and outcome of hospital-treated head injury in Rhode Island. *American Journal of Public Health, 76*(7), 773–778.

Fisher, B. A. (1980). *Small group decision making* (2nd ed.). New York: McGraw-Hill Book Company.

Fisher, J. M. (1985). Cognitive and behavioral consequences of closed head injury. *Seminars in Neurology, 5,* 3–8.

Fordyce, D. J., & Roueche, J. R. (1986). Changes in perspectives of disability among patients, staff, and relatives during rehabilitation of brain injury. *Rehabilitation Psychology, 31,* 217–229.

Fordyce, D. J., Roueche, J. R., & Prigatano, G. P. (1983). Enhanced emotional reactions in chronic head trauma patients. *Journal of Neurology, Neurosurgery, and Psychiatry, 46,* 620–624.

Frankowski, R. F., Annegers J. F., & Whitman S. (1985). Epidemiological and descriptive studies, part I: The descriptive epidemiology of head trauma in the United States. In D. P. Becker & J. T. Povlishock (Eds.), *Central nervous system trauma status report* (pp. 33–43). Bethesda, MD: National Institute of Neurological and Communicative Disorders and Stroke, National Institutes of Health.

Frederiksen, C. H., Bracewell, R. J., Breuleux, A., & Renaud, A. (1990). The cognitive representation and processing of discourse: Function and dysfunction. In Y. Joanette & H. H. Brownell (Eds.), *Discourse ability and brain damage: Theoretical and empirical perspectives* (pp. 69–110). New York: Springer-Verlag.

Freeman, M. R., Mittenberg, W., Dicowden, M., & Bat–Ami, M. (1992). Executive and compensatory memory retraining in traumatic brain injury. *Brain Injury, 6,* 65–70.

Fugl-Meyer, A. R., Branholm, I-B., & Fugl-Meyer K. S. (1991). Happiness and domain-specific life satisfaction in adult northern Swedes. *Clinical Rehabilitation, 5,* 25–33.

Gallagher, T. M. (1991). Language and social skills: Implications for assessment and intervention with school-age children. In T. M. Gallagher (Ed.), *Pragmatics of language: Clinical practice issues* (pp. 11–41). San Diego: Singular Publishing Group.

Gajar, A., Schloss, P. J., Schloss, C. N., & Thompson, C. K. (1984). Effects of feedback and self-monitoring on head trauma youths' conversation skills. *Journal of Applied Behavior Analysis, 17,* 353–358.

Garrison, J. W. (1986). Some principles of postpositivistic philosophy of science. *Educational Researcher, 15,* 12–15.

Gennarelli, T. A., Thibault, L. E., Adams, J. H., Graham, D. I., Thompson, C. J., & Marcincin, R. P. (1982). Diffuse axonal injury and traumatic coma in the primate. *Annals of Neurology, 12,* 564–574.

German, D. J. (1987). Spontaneous language profiles of children with word-finding problems. *Language, Speech, and Hearing Services in Schools, 18,* 217–230.

Gianutsos, R., & Matheson, P. (1987). The rehabilitation of visual perceptual disorders attributable to brain injury. In M. Meier, A. Benton, & L. Diller (Eds.), *Neuropsychological rehabilitation* (pp. 202–241). New York: The Guilford Press.

Gilchrist, E., & Wilkinson, M. (1979). Some factors determining prognosis in young people with severe head injuries. *Archives of Neurology, 36,* 355–358.

Giles, G. M., & Clark-Wilson, J. (1993). *Brain injury rehabilitation: A neurofunctional approach.* San Diego: Singular Publishing Group.

Giles, G., Fussey, I., & Burgess, P. (1988). The behavioral treatment of verbal interaction skills following severe head injury: A single case study. *Brain Injury, 2,* 75–79.

Glang, A., Singer, G., Cooley, E., & Tish, N. (1992). Tailoring direct instruction techniques for use with elementary students with brain injury. *Journal of Head Trauma Rehabilitation, 7*(4), 93–108.

Glosser, G., & Deser, T. (1990). Patterns of discourse production among neurological patients with fluent language disorders. *Brain and Language, 40,* 67–88.

Gobble, E. M. R., Henry, K., Pfahl, J. C., & Smith, G. J. (1987). Work adjustment services. In M. Ylvisaker & E. M. R. Gobble (Eds.), *Community re-entry for head injured adults* (pp. 221–258). Austin, TX: Pro-Ed.

Godfrey, H. P. D., Knight, R. G., Marsh, N. V., Moroney, B. M., & Bishara, S. N. (1989). Social interaction and speed of information processing following very severe closed head injury. *Psychological Medicine, 19,* 175–183.

Golden, C. J. (1978). *Stroop Color and Word Test.* Chicago: Stoelting Company.

Goldman-Rakic, P. S. (1993). Specification of higher cortical functions. *Journal of Head Trauma Rehabilitation, 8*(1), 13–23.

Goldstein, A., Sprafkin, R., Gershaw, N., & Klein, P. (1980). *Skill-streaming the adolescent.* Champaign, IL: Research Press.

Goldstein, F. C., & Levin, H. S. (1987). Disorders of reasoning and problem-solving ability. In M. Meier, A. Benton, & L. Diller (Eds.), *Neuropsychological rehabilitation* (pp. 327–354). New York: The Guilford Press.

Goodglass, H., and Kaplan, E. (1983). *Boston Diagnostic Aphasia Examination.* Philadelphia: Lea and Febiger.

Gordon, W. A., & Hibbard, M. R. (1991). The theory and practice of cognitive remediation. In J. S. Kreutzer & P. H. Wehman (Eds.), *Cognitive rehabilitation for persons with traumatic brain injury: A functional approach* (pp. 13–22). Baltimore: Paul H. Brookes Publishing.

Graesser, A. C. (1978). How to catch a fish: The memory and representation of common procedures. *Discourse Processes, 1*, 72–89.

Graesser, A. C. (1981). *Prose comprehension beyond the word.* New York: Springer-Verlag.

Grafman, J., Sirigu, A., Spector, L., & Hendler, J. (1993). Damage to the prefrontal cortex leads to decomposition of structure event complexes. *Journal of Head Trauma Rehabilitation, 8*(1), 73–87.

Graham, D. I., Adams, J. H., & Doyle, D. (1978). Ischemic brain damage in fatal nonmissile head injuries. *Journal of Neurological Sciences, 39*, 213–234.

Graham, D. I., Adams, J. H., & Gennarelli, T. A. (1987). Pathology of brain damage in head injury. In P. R. Cooper (Ed.), *Head injury* (2nd ed., pp. 72–88). New York: Williams and Wilkins.

Granger, C. V., Hamilton, B. B., & Kayton, R. (1986). *Uniform data system for medical rehabilitation.* Buffalo: Research Foundation, State University of New York.

Grice, H. (1975). Logic and conversation. In P. Cole & J. Morgan (Eds.), *Studies in syntax and semantics: Vol. 3. Speech acts* (pp. 41–58). New York: Academic Press.

Groher, M. (1990). Communication disorders in adults. In M. Rosenthal, E. R. Griffith, M. C. Bond, & J. D. Miller (Eds.), *Rehabilitation of the adult and child with traumatic brain injury* (2nd ed., pp. 148–162). Philadelphia: F. A. Davis.

Groher, M. E., & Ochipa, C. (1992). The standardized communication assessment of individuals with traumatic brain injury. *Seminars in Speech and Language, 13*, 252–263.

Gronwall, D. M. A. (1977). Paced auditory serial addition task: A measure of recovery from concussion. *Perceptual and Motor Skills, 44*, 367–373.

Gronwall, D. M. A. (1987). Advances in the assessment of attention and information processing after head injury. In H. S. Levin, J. Grafman, & H. M. Eisenberg (Eds.), *Neurobehavioral recovery from head injury* (pp. 355–371). New York: Oxford University Press.

Gronwall, D. M. A., & Sampson, H. (1974). *The psychological effects of concussion.* Auckland, New Zealand: Auckland University Press.

Gross, Y., & Schutz, L. E. (1986). Intervention models in neuropsychology. In B. P. Uzzell & Y. Gross (Eds.), *Clinical neuropsychology of intervention* (pp. 179–204). Boston: Martinus Nijhoff Publishing.

Gruen, A. K., Frankle, B. C., & Schwartz, R. (1990). Word fluency generation skills of head-injured patients in an acute trauma center. *Journal of Communication Disorders, 23*, 163–170.

Gualtieri, C. T. (1988). Pharmacotherapy and the neurobehavioural sequelae of traumatic brain injury. *Brain Injury, 2*, 101–129.

Haarbauer-Krupa, J., Henry, K., Szekeres, S. F., & Ylvisaker, M. (1985). Cognitive rehabilitation therapy: Late stages of recovery. In M. Ylvisaker (Ed.), *Head injury rehabilitation: Children and adolescents* (pp. 311–346). Austin, TX: Pro-Ed.

Haarbauer-Krupa, J., Moser, L., Smith, G. J., Sullivan, D. M. & Szekeres, S. F. (1985). Cognitive rehabilitation therapy: Middle stages of recovery. In M. Ylvisaker (Ed.), *Head injury rehabilitation: Children and adolescents* (pp. 287–310). Austin, TX: Pro-Ed.

Haas, J. F., Cope, D. N., & Hall, K. (1987). Premorbid prevalence of poor academic performance in severe head injury. *Journal of Neurology, Neurosurgery and Psychiatry, 50*, 52–56.

Hagen, C. (1984). Language disorders in head trauma. In A. Holland (Ed.), *Language disorders in adults: Recent advances.* (pp. 245–281). San Diego: College-Hill Press.

Hagen, C., & Malkmus, D. (1979, November). *Intervention strategies for language disorders secondary to head trauma.* American Speech-Language-Hearing Association Convention Short Course, Atlanta.

Hahn, S., & Klein, E. (1989). *Focus on function.* Tucson, AZ: Communication Skills Builders.

Halliday, M., & Hasan, R. (1976). *Cohesion in English.* London: Longman.

Halper, A. S., Cherney, L. R., & Miller, T. K. (1991). *Clinical management of communication problems in adults with traumatic brain injury.* Gaithersburg, MD: Aspen Publishers.

Hamilton, H. E. (1991). Accommodation and mental disability. In H. Giles, J. Coupland, & N. Coupland (Eds.), *Contexts of accommodation: Developments in applied sociolinguistics* (pp. 157–186). New York: Cambridge University Press.

Hammill, D. D. (1985). *Detroit Tests of Learning Aptitude (DTLA-2).* Austin, TX: Pro-Ed.

Hannay, J. H., & Levin, H. S. (1985). Selective reminding test: An examination of the equivalence of four forms. *Journal of Clinical and Experimental Neuropsychology, 7*, 251–263.

Hardman, J. M. (1979). The pathology of traumatic brain injuries. *Advances in Neurology, 22*, 15–50.

Harrison, C. L., & Dijkers M. (1992). Traumatic brain injury registries in the United States: An overview. *Brain Injury, 6*, 203–212.

Hart, T., & Hayden, M. E. (1986). The ecological validity of neuropsychological assessment and remediation. In B. P. Uzzell & Y. Gross (Eds.), *Clinical neuropsychology of intervention* (pp. 21–50). Boston: Martinus Nijhoff Publishing.

Hart, T., & Jacobs, H. E. (1993). Rehabilitation and management of behavioral disturbances following frontal lobe injury. *Journal of Head Trauma Rehabilitation, 8*(1), 1–12.

Hartley, L. (1986, November). Syntactic abilities of closed head injured patients in narrative discourse. Technical paper presented at 1986 American Speech-Language-Hearing Association National Convention, Detroit.

Hartley, L. (1990). Assessment of functional communication. In D. E. Tupper & K. D. Cicerone (Eds.), *The neuropsychology of everyday life, Volume 1: Assessment and basic competencies* (pp. 125–167). Boston: Kluwer Academic Publishers.

Hartley, L., & Griffith, A. (1988). A functional approach to the cognitive-communication deficits of closed head-injured clients. *Tejas: Texas Journal of Audiology and Speech Pathology, 14*(2), 37–42.

Hartley, L., & Jensen, P. J. (1991). Narrative and procedural discourse after closed head injury. *Brain Injury, 5*, 267–285.

Hartley, L., & Jensen, P. J. (1992). Three discourse profiles of closed-head-injury speakers: Theoretical and clinical implications. *Brain Injury, 6*, 271–281.

Hartley, L., & Levin, H. S. (1990). Linguistic deficits after closed head injury: A current appraisal. *Aphasiology, 4*, 353–370.

Haut, M. W., Petros, T. V., & Frank, R. G. (1990). The recall of prose as a function of importance following closed head injury. *Brain Injury, 4*, 281–288.

Haut, M. W., Petros, T. V., Frank, R. G., & Haut, J. S. (1991). Speed of processing within semantic memory following severe closed head injury. *Brain and Cognition, 17*, 31–41.

Heaton, R. K. (1981). *A manual for the Wisconsin Card Sorting Test*. Odessa, FL: Psychological Assessment Resources.

Helffenstein, D., & Wechsler, F. (1982). The use of interpersonal process recall in the remediation of interpersonal and communication skill deficits in the newly brain-injured. *Clinical Neuropsychology, 4*, 139–143.

Hensley, K. (1988). *Head injury program central registry statistics, state fiscal year 87/ 88 (July 1987–June 1988)*. Tallahassee: Florida Department of Labor and Employment Security, Division of Vocational Rehabilitation.

Hill, J., & Carper, M. (1985). Greenery: Group therapeutic approaches with the head injured. *Cognitive Rehabilitation, 3*(1), 18–28.

Hinkeldey, N. S., & Corrigan, J. D. (1990). The structure of head–injured patients' neurobehavioural complaints: A preliminary study. *Brain Injury, 4*, 115–134.

Holland, A. (1980). *Communicative Abilities in Daily Living*. Baltimore: University Park Press.

Holland, A. L. (1982). When is aphasia aphasia? The problem of closed head injury. In R. H. Brookshire (Ed.), *Clinical aphasiology: Conference proceedings* (pp. 345–349). Minneapolis: BRK Publishers.

Holland, S., & Ward, C. (1990). *Assertiveness: A practical approach*. Bichester, Great Britain: Winslow Press.

Hooper, H. E. (1958). *The Hooper Visual Organization Test: Manual*. Beverly Hills: Western Psychological Services.

Hooper Visual Organization Test (VOT). 1983 edition. Manual. Los Angeles: Western Psychological Services.

Horowitz, R., & Samuels, S. J. (1987). Comprehending oral and written language: Critical contrasts for literacy and schooling. In R. Horowitz & S. J. Samuels (Eds.), *Comprehending oral and written language* (pp. 1–52). New York: Academic Press.

Howe, J. R., & Miller, C. A. (1975). Midbrain deafness following head injury. *Neurology, 91*, 50–60.

Hux, K., Beukelman, D. R., Dombrovskis, M., & Snyder, R. (1993). Semantic organization following traumatic brain injury. *Journal of Medical Speech-Language Pathology, 1*, 121–131.

Interagency Head Injury Task Force. (1989). *Interagency Head Injury Task Force Report*. Washington, DC: U.S. Department of Health and Human Services, Public Health Service.

Jacobs, H. E. (1988). The Los Angeles head injury survey: Procedures and initial findings. *Archives of Physical Medicine and Rehabilitation, 69,* 425–431.

Jacobs, H. E. (1993). *Behavior analysis guidelines and brain injury rehabilitation: People, principles and programs.* Gaithersburg, MD: Aspen Publishers.

Jagger, J., Levine, J., & Jane, J. (1984). Epidemiologic features of head injury in a predominantly rural population. *Journal of Trauma, 24,* 40–44.

Joanette, Y., & Brownell, H. H. (Eds). (1990). *Discourse ability and brain damage: Theoretical and empirical perspectives.* New York: Springer-Verlag.

Johnson, D. A., & Newton, A. (1987). Social adjustment and interaction after severe head injury: II. Rationale and bases for intervention. *British Journal of Clinical Psychology, 26,* 289–298.

Jones-Gotman, M., & Milner, B. (1977). Design fluency: The invention of nonsense drawings after focal cortical lesion. *Neuropsychologia, 15,* 653–674.

Jorgenson, C., Barrett, M., Huisingh, R., & Zachman, L. (1981). *The Word Test.* Moline, IL: LinguiSystems.

Kaplan, E. (1988). A process approach to neuropsychological assessment. In T. Boll & B. K. Bryant (Eds.), *Clinical neuropsychology and brain function: Research, measurement, and practice* (pp. 129–167). Washington, DC: American Psychological Association.

Kaplan, E., Goodglass, H., & Weintraub, S. (1983). *The Boston Naming Test.* Philadelphia: Lea and Febiger.

Kaplan, S. P. (1991). Psychosocial adjustment three years after traumatic brain injury. *The Clinical Neuropsychologist, 4,* 360–369.

Katz, R., LaPointe, L., & Markel, N. (1978). Coverbal behavior and aphasic speakers. In R. Brookshire (Ed.), *Clinical aphasiology conference proceedings* (pp. 164–173). Minneapolis: BRK Publishers.

Kay, T., Cavallo, M. M., & Ezrachi, O. (1988). *Administration manual, N.Y.U. Head Injury Family Interview (Version 1.2).* New York: Research and Training Center on Head Trauma and Stroke.

Kearns, K. P. (1989). Methodologies for studying generalization. In L. McReynolds & J. E. Spradlin (Eds.), *Generalization strategies in the treatment of communication disorders* (pp. 13–30). Philadelphia: B. C. Decker.

Kellermann, K., Broetzmann, S., Lim, T., & Kitao, K. (1989). The conversation mop: Scenes in the stream of discourse. *Discourse Processes, 12,* 27–61.

Kennedy, M., & DeRuyter, F. (1991). Cognitive and language bases for communication disorders. In D. Beukelman & K. Yorkston (Eds.), *Communication disorders following traumatic brain injury: Management of cognitive, language, and motor impairments* (pp. 123–190). Austin, TX: Pro-Ed.

Kertesz, A. (1982). *Western Aphasia Battery.* New York: Grune & Stratton.

Kewman, D. G., Yanus, B., & Kirsch, N. (1988). Assessment of distractibility in auditory comprehension after traumatic brain injury. *Brain Injury, 2,* 131–137.

Kløve, H. (1987). Activation, arousal, and neuropsychological rehabilitation. *Journal of Clinical and Experimental Neuropsychology, 9,* 297–309.

Kneipp, S., & Paul-Cohen, R. (1993). Community-based services and support for individuals with traumatic brain injury. *Seminars in Speech and Language, 14,* 32–43.

Koegel, L. K., Koegel, R. L., & Ingham, J. C. (1986). Programming rapid generalization of correct articulation through self-monitoring procedures. *Journal of Speech and Hearing Disorders, 51,* 24–32.

Kozloff, R. (1987). Networks of social support and the outcome from severe head injury. *Journal of Head Trauma Rehabilitation, 2*(3), 14–23.

Kraus, J. F. (1987). Epidemiology of head injury. In P. R. Cooper (Ed.), *Head injury* (2nd ed.) (pp. 1–19). New York: Williams and Wilkins.

Kreutzer, J. S., Camplair, P., & Waaland, P. (1988). *Family needs questionnaire.* Richmond: Medical College of Virginia, Rehabilitation Research and Training Center on Severe Traumatic Brain Injury.

Kreutzer, J. S., Devany, C. W., Myers, S. L., & Marwitz, J. H. (1991). Neurobehavioral outcome following traumatic brain injury: Review, methodology, and implications for cognitive rehabilitation. In J. S. Kreutzer & P. H. Wehman (Eds.), *Cognitive rehabilitation for persons with traumatic brain injury: A functional approach* (pp. 55–74). Baltimore: Paul H. Brookes Publishing Co.

Kreutzer, J. S., Leininger, B. E., Doherty, K., & Waaland, P. K. (1987). *General health and history questionnaire.* Richmond: Medical College of Virginia, Rehabilitation Research and Training Center on Severe Brain Injury.

Kreutzer, J. S., Leininger, B. E., & Harris, J. A. (1990). The evolving role of neuropsychology in community integration. In J. S. Kreutzer & P. Wehman (Eds.), *Community integration following traumatic brain injury* (pp. 49–66). Baltimore: Paul H. Brookes Publishing Co.

Kreutzer, J. S., & Wehman, P. (1990). *Community integration following traumatic brain injury.* Baltimore: Paul H. Brookes Publishing Co.

Kreutzer, J. S., Wehman, P., Morton, M. V., & Stonnington, H. H. (1988). Supported employment and compensatory strategies for enhancing vocational outcome following traumatic brain injury. *Brain Injury, 2,* 205–223.

Labov, W. (1972). *Language in the inner city.* Philadelphia: University of Pennsylvania Press.

Lal, S., Merbtiz, C. P., & Grip, J. C. (1988). Modification of function in head–injured patients with Sinemet. *Brain Injury, 2*(3), 225–233.

Lam, C., McMahon, B., Priddy, D., & Gehred-Schultze, A. (1988). Deficit awareness and treatment performance among traumatic head injury adults. *Brain Injury, 2,* 235–242.

Larson, C., Backlund, P., Redmond, M., & Barbour, A. (1978). *Assessing functional communication.* Annandale, VA: Speech Communication Association.

Lawson, M. J., & Rice, D. N. (1989). Effects of training in use of executive strategies on a verbal memory problem resulting from closed head injury. *Journal of Clinical and Experimental Neuropsychology, 11,* 842–854.

Lehmkuhl, L. D., Kreutzer, J. S., & Gordan, W. A. (1992, December). *Multicenter collaboration: Summary of findings of the TBI model systems.* Presentation at the Annual Symposium of the National Head Injury Foundation, Boston.

Lennox, D. B., & Brune, P. (1993). Incidental teaching for training communication in individuals with traumatic brain injury. *Brain Injury, 5,* 449–454.

Levin, H. S., Eisenberg, H., & Benton, A. L. (Eds.). (1991). *Frontal lobe function and dysfunction.* New York: Oxford University Press.

Levin, H. S., & Goldstein, F. C. (1986). Organization of verbal memory after severe closed-head injury. *Journal of Clinical and Experimental Neuropsychology, 8*, 643–656.

Levin, H. S., Grafman, J., & Eisenberg, H. M. (Eds.). (1987). *Neurobehavioral recovery from head injury.* New York: Oxford University Press.

Levin, H. S., Grossman, R. G., Rose, J. E., & Teasdale, G. (1979). Long-term neuropsychological outcome of closed head injury. *Journal of Neurosurgery, 50*, 412–422.

Levin, H. S., Grossman, R. G., Sarwar, M., & Meyers, C. A. (1981). Linguistic recovery after closed head injury. *Brain and Language, 12*, 360–374.

Levin, H. S., High, W. M., Goethe, K., Sisson, R. A., Overall, J., Rhoades, H., Eisenberg, H. M., Kalisky, Z., & Gary, H. (1987). The Neurobehavioral Rating Scale: Assessment of the behavioral sequelae of head injury by the clinician. *Journal of Neurology, Neurosurgery, and Psychiatry, 50*, 183–193.

Levin, H. S., O'Donnell, V. M., & Grossman, R. G. (1979). The Galveston Orientation and Amnesia Test: A practical scale to assess cognition after head injury. *Journal of Nervous and Mental Diseases, 167*, 675–684.

Levinson, S. C. (1983). *Pragmatics.* Cambridge, England: Cambridge University Press.

Lewis, F. D., & Bitter, C. F. (1991). Applied behavior analysis and work adjustment training. In B. T. McMahon & L. R. Shaw (Eds.), *Work worth doing: Advances in brain injury rehabilitation* (pp. 137–164). Winter Park, FL: PMD Press, Inc.

Lewis, F. D., Nelson, J., Nelson, C., & Reusink, P. (1988). Effects of three feedback contingencies on the socially inappropriate talk of a brain–injured adult. *Behavior Therapy, 19*, 203–211.

Lezak, M. D. (1978). Living with the characterologically altered brain injured patient. *Journal of Clinical Psychiatry, 39*, 592–598.

Lezak, M. D. (1982). The problem of assessing executive functions. *International Journal of Psychology, 17*, 281–297.

Lezak, M. D. (1983). *Neuropsychological assessment* (2nd ed.). New York: Oxford University Press.

Lezak, M. D. (1987a). Assessment for rehabilitation planning. In M. Meier, A. Benton, & L. Diller (Eds.), *Neuropsychological rehabilitation* (pp. 41–58). New York: The Guilford Press.

Lezak, M. D. (1987b). Relationships between personality disorders, social disturbances, and physical disability following traumatic brain injury. *Journal of Head Trauma Rehabilitation, 2*(1), 57–69.

Lezak, M. D. (1989). Assessment of psychological dysfunctions resulting from head trauma. In M. D. Lezak (Ed.), *Assessment of the behavioral consequences of head trauma* (pp. 113–143). New York: Alan R. Liss.

Lezak, M. D. (1993). Newer contributions to the neuropsychological assessment of executive functions. *Journal of Head Trauma Rehabilitation, 8*(1), 24–31.

Liberman, R. P., (1982). Assessment of social skills. *Schizophrenia Bulletin, 8*, 62–83.

Liberman, R. P., King, L. W., DeRisi, W. J., & McCann, M. (1975). *Personal effectiveness: Guiding people to assert themselves and improve their social skills.* Champaign, IL: Research Press.

Liberman, R. P., DeRisi, W. J., & Mueser, K. T. (1989). *Social skills training for psychiatric patients.* Needham Heights, MA: Allyn and Bacon.

Likert, R. (1961). *New patterns of management.* New York: McGraw-Hill.

Likert, R. (1967). *The human organization.* New York: McGraw-Hill.

Liles, B. Z., Coelho, C. A., Duffy, R. J., & Zalagens, M. R. (1989). Effects of elicitation procedures on the narratives of normal and closed head-injured adults. *Journal of Speech and Hearing Disorders, 54*, 356–366.

Loban, W. (1976). *Language development: Kindergarten through grade twelve.* Urbana, IL: National Council of Teachers of English.

Lundsteen, S. (1979). *Listening.* Urbana, IL: National Council of Teachers of English.

Luria, A. (1973). *The working brain: An introduction to neuropsychology* (B. Haigh, Trans.). New York: Basic Books.

MacNiven, E., & Finlayson, M. A. J. (1993). The interplay between emotional and cognitive recovery after closed head injury. *Brain Injury, 7*, 241–246.

Malkmus, D. D. (1989). Community reentry: Cognitive-communicative intervention within a social skill context. *Topics in Language Disorders, 9*(2), 50–66.

Malec, J. (1984). Training the brain-injured client in behavioral self-management skills. In B. A. Edelstein & E. T. Couture (Eds.), *Behavioral assessment and rehabilitation of the traumatically brain-damaged* (pp. 121–150). New York: Plenum Press.

Marquardt, T. P., Stoll, J., & Sussman, H. (1990). Disorders of communication in traumatic brain injury. In E. D. Bigler (Ed.), *Traumatic brain injury: Mechanisms of damage, assessment, intervention, and outcome.* (pp. 181–205). Austin, TX: Pro-Ed.

Marsh, N. V., & Knight, R. G. (1991). Behavioral assessment of social competence following severe head injury. *Journal of Clinical and Experimental Neuropsychology, 13*, 729–740.

Marshall, R. (1976). Word retrieval behavior of aphasic adults. *Journal of Speech and Hearing Disorders, 41*, 444–451.

Martzke, J., Swan, C., & Varney, N. (1991). Post traumatic anosmia and orbital frontal damage: Neuropsychological and neuropsychiatric correlates. *Neuropsychology, 5*, 213–225.

Mateer, C. A., & Sohlberg, M. M. (1988). A paradigm shift in memory rehabilitation. In H. Whitaker (Ed.), *Neuropsychological studies of nonfocal brain damage: Dementia and trauma* (pp. 204–219). New York: Springer-Verlag.

Mateer, C. A., & Sohlberg, M. M. (1992). Process-oriented approaches to treatment of attention and memory disorders following traumatic brain injury. *Seminars in Speech and Language, 13*, 280–292.

Mateer, C. A., Sohlberg, M. M., & Crinean, J. (1987). Perceptions of memory functions in individuals with closed head injury. *Journal of Head Trauma Rehabilitation, 2*, 74–84.

Mateer, C. A., Sohlberg, M. M., & Youngman, P. K. (1990). The management of acquired attention and memory deficits. In R. L. Wood & I. Fussey (Eds.), *Cognitive rehabilitation in perspective* (pp. 68–96). New York: Taylor and Francis.

Mattson, A. J., & Levin, H. S. (1990). Frontal lobe dysfunction following closed head injury. *The Journal of Nervous and Mental Disorders, 178,* 282–291.

McCombs, B. L. (1988). Motivational skills training: Combining metacognitive, cognitive, and affective learning strategies. In C. E. Weinstein, E. T. Goetz, & P. A. Alexander (Eds.), *Learning and study strategies: Issues in assessment, instruction, and evaluation* (pp. 141–169). San Diego: Academic Press.

McLaughlin, A. M., & Carey, J. L. (1993). The adversarial alliance: Developing therapeutic relationships between families and the team in brain injury rehabilitation. *Brain Injury, 7,* 45–52.

McKinlay, W. W., Brooks, D. N., Bond, M., Martinage, D. P., & Marshall, M. M. (1981). The short–term outcome of severe blunt head injury as reported by relatives of the injured persons. *Journal of Neurology, Neurosurgery and Psychiatry, 44,* 527–533.

McNeil, J. D. (1992). *Reading comprehension: New directions for classroom practice* (3rd ed.). Los Angeles: HarperCollins.

McNeil, M. R., & Prescott, T. E. (1978). *Revised Token Test.* Baltimore: University Park Press.

McNeny, R., & Wilcox, P. (1991). Partners by force: The family and the rehabilitation team. *NeuroRehabilitation, 1(2),* 7–17.

McReynolds, L. V. (1989). Generalization issues in the treatment of communication disorders. In L. V. McReynolds & J. E. Spradlin (Eds.), *Generalization strategies in the treatment of communication disorders* (pp. 1–12). Philadelphia: B. C. Decker.

McTear, M. (1985). Pragmatic disorders: A case study of conversational disability. *British Journal of Disorders of Communication, 20,* 129–142.

McTear, M. F., & Conti-Ramsden, G. (1992). *Pragmatic disability in children.* San Diego: Singular Publishing Group.

Mehrabian, A. (1968). Communication without words. *Psychology Today, 2,* 51–52.

Meichenbaum, D. (1993). The "potential" contributions of cognitive behavior modification to the rehabilitation of individuals with traumatic brain injury. *Seminars in Speech and Language, 14,* 18–31.

Mentis, M., & Prutting, C. A. (1987). Cohesion in the discourse of normal and head-injured adults. *Journal of Speech and Hearing Research, 30,* 88–98.

Mentis, M., & Prutting, C. A. (1991). Analysis of topic as illustrated in a head-injured and a normal adult. *Journal of Speech and Hearing Research, 34,* 583–596.

Milton, S. (1985). Compensatory memory strategy training. *Cognitive Rehabilitation, 3(6),* 8–15.

Milton, S. (1988). Management of subtle cognitive communication deficits. *Journal of Head Trauma Rehabilitation, 3(2),* 1–11.

Milton, S., Prutting, C., & Binder, G. (1984). Appraisal of communicative competence in head injured adults. In R. Brookshire (Ed.), *Clinical aphasiology conference proceedings* (pp. 114–123). Minneapolis: BRK Publishers.

Milton, S., & Wertz, R. (1986). Management of persisting communication deficits in patients with traumatic brain injury. In B. Uzzell & Y. Gross (Eds.), *Clinical neuropsychology of intervention* (pp. 223–256). Boston: Martinus Nijhoff Publishing.

Moffat, N. (1984). Strategies of memory therapy. In B. A. Wilson & N. Moffat (Eds.), *Clinical management of memory problems*. London: Croom Helm.

Moore, A. D., Stambrook, M., & Peters, L. C. (1989). Coping strategies and adjustment after closed-head injury: A cluster analytical approach. *Brain Injury, 3*, 171–176.

Moruzzi, G., & Magoun, H. W. (1949). Brainstem reticular formation and activation of the EEG. *Electroencephalography and Clinical Neurophysiology, 1*, 455–473.

Murphy, C., & Jenks, L. (1982). *Getting a job—What skills are needed?* San Francisco: Far West Laboratory for Educational Research and Development.

Murphy, G. L. (1990). The psycholinguistics of discourse comprehension. In Y. Joanette & H. H. Brownell (Eds.), *Discourse ability and brain damage: Theoretical and empirical perspectives* (pp. 29–49). New York: Springer-Verlag.

Nagi, S. (1969). *Disability and rehabilitation: Legal, clinical, and self-concepts and measurements.* Columbus: Ohio State University Press.

Nelson, R. O., & Hayes, S. C. (1981). Theoretical explanations for reactivity in self-monitoring. *Behavior Modification, 5*, 3–14.

Newton, A., & Johnson, D. (1985). Social adjustment and interaction after severe head injury. *British Journal of Clinical Psychology, 24*, 225–234.

Noble, J. H., Conley, R. W., Laski, F., & Noble, M. A. (1990). Issues and problems in the treatment of traumatic brain injury. *Journal of Disability Policy Studies, 1*(2), 19–45.

Oddy, M. (1984). Head injury and social adjustment. In N. Brooks (Ed.), *Closed head injury: Psychological, social, and family consequences* (pp. 108–192). New York: Oxford University Press.

Oddy, M., Coughlan, T., Tyerman, A., & Jenkins, D. (1985). Social adjustment after closed head injury: A further follow up seven years after injury. *Journal of Neurology, Neurosurgery and Psychiatry, 48*, 564–568.

Oddy, M., & Humphrey, M. (1980). Social recovery during the year following severe head injury. *Journal of Neurology, Neurosurgery, and Psychiatry, 43*, 798–802.

Oddy, M., Humphrey, M., & Uttley, D. (1978). Stresses upon the relatives of head-injured patients. *British Journal of Psychiatry, 133*, 507–513.

O'Hara, C. C., & Harrell, M. (1991). *Rehabilitation with brain injury survivors: An empowerment approach.* Gaithersburg, MD: Aspen Publishers.

Ojemann, G. A. (1978). Organization of short-term verbal memory in language areas of human cortex: Evidence from electrical stimulation. *Brain and Language, 5*, 331–340.

Ommaya, A. K., & Gennarelli, T. A. (1974). Cerebral concussion and traumatic unconsciousness. *Brain, 97*, 633–654.

Orsillo, S. M., McCaffrey, R. J., & Fisher, J. (1993). Siblings of head-injured individuals: A population at risk. *Journal of Head Trauma Rehabilitation, 8*(1), 102–115.

O'Shanick, G. J., & Parmelee, D. X. (1989). Psychopharmacological agents in the treatment of brain injury. In D. W. Ellis & A. Christensen (Eds.), *Neuropsychological treatment after brain injury* (pp. 91–104). Boston: Kluwer Academic Publishers.

O'Shanick, G. J., & Zasler, N. D. (1990). Neuropsychopharmacological approaches to traumatic brain injury. In J. S. Kreutzer & P. Wehman (Eds.), *Community integration following traumatic brain injury* (pp. 15–28). Baltimore: Paul H. Brookes Publishing Co.

Painter, C. M. (1985). A survey of communication skills needed on-the-job by technical students. *Journal of Studies in Technical Careers*, 7, 153–160.

Pang, D. (1985). Pathophysiologic correlates of neurobehavioral syndromes following closed head injury. In M. Ylvisaker (Ed.), *Head injury rehabilitation: Children and adolescents* (pp. 3–70). Austin, TX: Pro-Ed.

Parenté, R., & Anderson-Parenté, J. K. (1989). Retraining memory: Theory and application. *The Journal of Head Trauma Rehabilitation*, 4(3), 55–65.

Parenté, R., & Anderson-Parenté, J. K. (1990). Vocational memory training. In J. S. Kreutzer & P. Wehman (Eds.), *Community integration following traumatic brain injury* (pp. 157–168). Baltimore: Paul H. Brookes Publishing Co.

Parenté, R., & DiCesare, A. (1991). Retraining memory: Theory, evaluation, and applications. In J. S. Kreutzer & P. H. Wehman (Eds.), *Cognitive rehabilitation for persons with traumatic brain injury: A functional approach* (pp. 147–162). Baltimore: Paul H. Brooks Publishing Co.

Pehrsson, R. S., & Denner, P. R. (1988). Semantic organizers: Implications for reading and writing. *Topics in Language Disorders*, 8, 24–37.

Penn, C., & Cleary, J. (1988). Compensatory strategies in the language of closed head injured patients. *Brain Injury*, 2, 3–17.

Peters, M. D., Gluck, M., & McCormick, M. (1992). Behaviour rehabilitation of the challenging client in less restrictive settings. *Brain Injury*, 6, 299–314.

Ponsford, J. L. (1990). Psychological sequelae of closed head injury: Time to redress the imbalance. *Brain Injury*, 4, 111–114.

Ponsford, J. L., & Kinsella, G. (1988). Evaluation of a remedial program for attentional deficits following closed-head injury. *Journal of Clinical and Experimental Neuropsychology*, 10, 693–708.

Ponsford, J., & Kinsella, G. (1992). Attentional deficits following closed-head injury. *Journal of Clinical and Experimental Neuropsychology*, 14, 822–838.

Porteus, S. D. (1959). *The Maze Test and clinical psychology*. Palo Alto, CA: Pacific Books.

Porteus, S. D. (1965). *Porteus Maze Test. Fifty years' application*. San Antonio, TX: The Psychological Corporation.

Posner, M. I., & Rafal, R. D. (1987). Cognitive theories of attention and the rehabilitation of attentional deficits. In M. Meier, A. Benton, & L. Diller (Eds.), *Neuropsychological rehabilitation* (pp. 182–201). New York: The Guilford Press.

Pressley, M. (1993). Teaching cognitive strategies to brain-injured clients: The good information processing perspective. *Seminars in Speech and Language*, 14, 1–17.

Pribram, K. H. (1971). *Languages of the brain: Experimental paradoxes and principles in neuropsychology* (2nd ed.). Englewood Cliffs, NJ: Prentice-Hall.

Prigatano, G. P. (1987). Personality and psychosocial consequences after brain injury. In M. Meier, A. Benton, & L. Diller (Eds.), *Neuropsychological rehabilitation* (pp. 355–378). New York: The Guilford Press.

Prigatano, G. P. (1989). Bring it up in milieu: Toward effective traumatic brain injury rehabilitation interaction. *Rehabilitation Psychology*, 34, 135–143.

Prigatano, G. P., Altman, I. M., & O'Brien, K. P. (1990). Behavioral limitations that traumatic brain-injured patients tend to underestimate. *The Clinical Neuropsychologist*, 4(2), 163–176.

Prigatano, G. P., Pepping, M., & Klonoff, P. (1986). Cognitive, personality and psychosocial factors in neuropsychological adjustment of brain-injured patients. In B. P. Uzzell & Y. Gross (Eds.), *Clinical neuropsychology of intervention* (pp. 135–166). Boston: Martinus Nijhoff.

Prigatano, G., Roueche, J., & Fordyce, D. (1986). Nonaphasic language disturbances after brain injury. In G. P. Prigatano (Ed.), *Neuropsychological rehabilitation after brain injury* (pp. 18–28). Baltimore: Johns Hopkins University Press.

Prutting, C. (1982). Pragmatics as social competence. *Journal of Speech and Hearing Disorders, 47,* 123–133.

Prutting, C., & Kirchner, D. (1983). Applied pragmatics. In T. Gallagher & C. Prutting (Eds.), *Pragmatic assessment and intervention issues in language* (pp. 29–64). San Diego: College-Hill Press.

Prutting, C., & Kirchner, D. (1987). A clinical appraisal of the pragmatic aspects of language. *Journal of Speech and Hearing Disorders, 52,* 105–119.

Quick, J. C., Nelson, D. L., & Quick, J. D. (1990). *Stress and challenge at the top: The paradox of the successful executive.* New York: John Wiley.

Quick, J. C., & Quick, J. D. (1984). *Organizational stress and preventive management.* New York: McGraw-Hill.

Ramsberger, G. (1994). Functional perspective for assessment and rehabilitation of persons with severe aphasia. *Seminars in Speech and Language, 15*(1), 1–16.

Ratcliff, G. (1987). Perception and complex visual processes. In M. Meier, A. Benton, & L. Diller (Eds.), *Neuropsychological rehabilitation* (pp. 242–259). New York: The Guilford Press.

Reitan, R. M. (1958). Validity of the Trail Making Test as an indication of organic brain damage. *Perceptual and Motor Skills, 8,* 271–276.

Reitan, R. M. & Wolfson, D. (1985). *The Halstead Reitan Neuropsychological Test Battery.* Tuscon, AZ: Neuropsychology Press.

Rey, A. (1941). L'examen psychologique dans les cas d'encephalopathie traumatique. *Archives de Psychologie, 28,* 286–340.

Rey, A. (1964). *L'examen clinique en psychologie.* Paris: Presses Universitaires de France.

Riccardi, V. M., & Kurtz, S. M. (1983). *Communication and counseling in health care.* Springfield, IL: Charles C Thomas.

Rimel, R. W., Giordani, B., Barth, J. T., Boll, T. J., & Jane, J. A. (1981). Disability caused by minor head injury. *Neurosurgery, 9,* 221–229.

Rimel, R. W., & Jane, J. A. (1984). Patient characteristics. In M. Rosenthal, E. R. Griffith, M. R. Bond & J. D. Miller (Eds.), *Rehabilitation of the head-injured adult* (pp. 9–20). Philadelphia: F. A. Davis.

Ripich, D. N., & Spinelli, F. M. (1985). An ethnographic approach to assessment and intervention. In D. N. Ripich & F. M. Spinelli (Eds.), *School discourse problems* (pp. 199–216). San Diego: Singular Publishing Group.

Ross, D. (1986). *Ross Information Processing Assessment.* Austin, TX: Pro-Ed.

Rost, M. (1990). *Listening in language learning.* New York: Longman.

Roth, F., & Spekman, N. (1984). Assessing the pragmatic abilities of children: Part I. Organizational framework and assessment parameters. *Journal of Speech and Hearing Disorders, 49,* 2–11.

Royer, J. M., & Cunningham, D. J. (1981). On the theory and measurement of reading comprehension. *Contemporary Educational Psychology, 6,* 187–216.

Ruff, R. M., Light, R. H., & Evans, R. W. (1987). The Ruff Figural Fluency Test: A normative study with adults. *Developmental Neuropsychology, 3*, 37-52.

Ruff, R. M., Niemann, H., Troster, A. I., & Mateer, C. A. (1990). Effectiveness of behavioral management in rehabilitation: Cognitive procedures. In R. L. Wood (Ed.), *Neurobehavioural sequelae of traumatic brain injury* (pp. 303-335). New York: Taylor and Francis.

Sacks, H., Schegloff, E., & Jefferson, G. (1974). A simplest systematics for the organization of turn-taking for conversation. *Language, 50*, 606-735.

Salcido, R., & Costich, J. F. (1992). Recurrent traumatic brain injury. *Brain Injury, 6*, 293-298.

Sampson, E. E., & Marthas, M. (1990). *Group process for the health professions* (3rd ed.). Albany, NY: Delmar Publishers.

Sarno, M. T. (1980). The nature of verbal impairment after closed head injury. *Journal of Nervous and Mental Disease, 11*, 685-692.

Sarno, M. T. (1984a). Functional measurement in verbal impairment secondary to brain damage. In C. Granger & G. Gresham (Eds.), *Functional assessment in rehabilitation medicine* (pp. 210-222). Baltimore: Williams and Wilkins.

Sarno, M. T. (1984b). Verbal impairment after closed head injury: Report of a replication study. *Journal of Nervous and Mental Disorders, 172*, 475-479.

Sarno, M. T. (1988). Language and speech defects. *Scandinavian Journal of Rehabilitation Medicine, 17*(Suppl.), 55-64.

Sarno, M. T., Buonaguro, A. & Levita, E. (1986). Characteristics of verbal impairment in closed head injury. *Archives of Physical Medicine and Rehabilitation, 67*, 400-405.

Sarno, M. T., & Levita, E. (1979). Recovery in treated aphasia in the first year post stroke. *Stroke, 10*, 663-670.

Sbordone, R. J. (1984). Rehabilitative neuropsychological approach for severe traumatic brain-injured patients. *Professional Psychology: Research and Practice, 15*, 165-175.

Sbordone, R. J. (1991). Overcoming obstacles in cognitive rehabilitation of persons with severe traumatic brain injury. In J. S. Kreutzer & P. H. Wehman (Eds.), *Cognitive rehabilitation for persons with traumatic brain injury: A functional approach* (pp. 105-116). Baltimore: Paul H. Brookes Publishing Company.

Schacter, D. L., & Glisky, E. L. (1986). Memory remediation: Restoration, alleviation, and the acquisition of domain-specific knowledge. In B. P. Uzzell & Y. Gross (Eds.), *Clinical neuropsychology of intervention* (pp. 257-282). Boston: Martinus Nijhoff.

Schank, R. C. (1982). *Dynamic memory: A theory of reminding and learning in computers and people.* Cambridge, England: Cambridge University Press.

Schank, R. C., & Abelson, R. (1977). *Scripts, plans, goals and understanding: An inquiry into human knowledge structures.* Hillsdale, NJ: Lawrence Erlbaum.

Schloss, P. J., Thompson, C. K., Gajar, A. H., & Schloss, C. N. (1985). Influence of self-monitoring on heterosexual conversational behaviors of head trauma youth. *Applied Research in Mental Retardation, 6*, 269-282.

Schmitter-Edgecombe, M., Marks, W., Fahy, J. F., & Long C. J. (1992). Effects of severe closed-head injury on three stages of information processing. *Journal of Clinical and Experimental Neuropsychology, 14*, 717-737.

Schuell, H. (1972). *Minnesota Test for Differential Diagnosis of Aphasia—Revised.* Minneapolis: University of Minnesota Press.

Schwartz, L., & McKinley, N. (1984). *Daily communication.* Eau Claire, WI: Thinking Publications.

Schwartz, M. F., Mayer, N. H., Fitzpatrick De Salme, E. J., & Montgomery, M.W. (1993). Cognitive theory and the study of everyday action disorders after brain damage. *Journal of Head Trauma Rehabilitation, 8*(1), 59–72.

Scinto, L. (1977). Textual competence: A preliminary analysis of orally generated texts. *Linguistics, 194,* 5–34.

Searle, J. R. (1969). *Speech acts.* London: Cambridge University Press.

Shallice, T. (1982). Specific impairments of planning. *Philosophical Transactions of the Royal Society of London, 298,* 199–209.

Shallice, T., & Burgess, P. (1991). Higher-order cognitive impairments and frontal lobe lesions in man. In H. S. Levin, H. M. Eisenberg, & A. L. Benton (Eds.), *Frontal lobe function and dysfunction* (pp. 125–138). New York: Oxford University Press.

Shaw, L. R., & McMahon, B. T. (1990). Family-staff conflict in the rehabilitation setting: Causes, consequences, and implications. *Brain Injury, 4,* 87–94.

Singer, G. H. S., & Powers, L. E. (1993). Contributing to resilience in families: An overview. In G. H. S. Singer, & L. E. Powers (Eds.), *Families, disability and empowerment: Active coping skills and strategies for family interventions* (pp. 1–25). Baltimore: Paul H. Brookes Publishing Co.

Singer, M. (1990). *Psychology of language: An introduction to sentence and discourse processes.* Hillsdale, NJ: Lawrence Erlbaum Associates.

Smith, A. (1973). *Symbol Digit Modalities Test.* Los Angeles: Western Psychological Services.

Smith, G. J., & Ylvisaker, M. (1985). Cognitive rehabilitation therapy: Early stages of recovery. In M. Ylvisaker (Ed.), *Head injury rehabilitation: Children and adolescents* (pp. 275–286). Austin, TX: Pro-Ed.

Sohlberg, M. M., & Mateer, C. A. (1987). Efficacy of an attention process training program. *Journal of Clinical and Experimental Neuropsychology, 9,* 117–130.

Sohlberg, M. M., & Mateer, C. A. (1989a). The assessment of cognitive-communicative functions in head injury. *Topics in Language Disorders, 9*(2), 15–33.

Sohlberg, M. M., & Mateer, C. A. (1989b). *Introduction to cognitive rehabilitation: Theory and practice.* New York: Guilford.

Sohlberg, M. M., & Mateer, C. A. (1989c). Training use of compensatory memory books: A three stage behavioral approach. *Journal of Clinical and Experimental Neuropsychology, 11,* 871–891.

Sohlberg, M. M., & Mateer, C. A. (1990). Evaluation and treatment of communicative skills. In J. S. Kreutzer & P. Wehman (Eds.), *Community integration following traumatic brain injury* (pp. 67–82). Baltimore: Paul H. Brookes Publishing Company.

Sohlberg, M. M., Mateer, C. A., & Stuss, D. T. (1993). Contemporary approaches to the management of executive control dysfunction. *Journal of Head Trauma Rehabilitation, 8*(1), 45–58.

Sohlberg, M. M., White, O., Evans, E., & Mateer, C. (1992a). Background and initial case studies into the effects of prospective memory training. *Brain Injury, 6,* 129–138.

Sohlberg, M. M., White, O., Evans, E., & Mateer, C. (1992b). An investigation of the effects of prospective memory training. *Brain Injury, 6,* 139–154.

Solomon, C. R., & Scherzer, B. P. (1991). Some guidelines for family therapists working with the traumatically brain injured and their families. *Brain Injury, 5,* 253–266.

Sparadeo, F. R., Strauss, D., & Barth, J. T. (1990). The incidence, impact, and treatment of substance abuse in head trauma rehabilitation. *Journal of Head Trauma Rehabilitation, 5*(3), 1–8.

Spitzberg, B. H. (1983). Communication competence as knowledge, skill, and impression. *Communication Education, 32,* 323–329.

Spitzberg, B. H., Brookshire, R. G., & Brunner, C. C. (1990). The factorial domain of interpersonal skills. *Social Behavior and Personality, 18,* 137–150.

Spitzberg, B. H., & Hurt, H. T. (1987). The measurement of interpersonal skills in instructional contexts. *Communication Education, 36,* 28–45.

Spitzberg, B. H., & Huwe, R. (1991, November). *Oral communication competency in interpersonal communication: The conversational skills rating scale.* Paper presented at the Speech Communication Association Conference, Atlanta.

Spreen, O., & Benton, A. L. (1977). *Neurosensory Center Comprehensive Examination for Aphasia-Revised.* Victoria, British Columbia: University of Victoria Neuropsychology Laboratory.

Spreen, O., & Strauss, E. (1991). *A compendium of neuropsychological tests: Administration, norms, and commentary.* New York: Oxford University Press.

Stein, N. L., & Glenn, C. G. (1979). An analysis of story comprehension in elementary school children. In R. O. Freedle (Ed.), *New directions in discourse processing II* (pp. 53–120). Norwood, NJ: Ablex.

Stokes, T. F., & Baer, D. M. (1977). An implicit technology of generalization. *Journal of Applied Behavior Analysis, 10,* 344–367.

Strich, S. J. (1969). The pathology of brain damage due to blunt head injuries. In A. E. Walker, W. F. Caveness, & M. Critchley (Eds.), *The late effects of head injury* (pp. 501–524). Springfield, IL: Charles C Thomas.

Stroop, J. R. (1935). Studies of interference in serial verbal reactions. *Journal of Experimental Psychology, 18,* 643–662.

Stuss, D. T. (1991). Self, awareness, and the frontal lobes: A neuropsychological perspective. In G. R. Goethaals & J. Strauss (Eds.), *The self: An interdisciplinary approach* (pp. 255–278). New York: Springer-Verlag.

Stuss, D. T., Delgado, M., & Guzman, D. A. (1987). Verbal regulation in the control of motor impersistence: A proposed rehabilitation procedure. *Journal of Neurological Rehabilitation, 1,* 19–24.

Symonds, C. (1937). Mental disorder following head injury. *Proceedings of the Royal Society Medicine, 30,* 1081–1094.

Szekeres, S. (1992). Organization as an intervention target after traumatic brain injury. *Seminars in Speech and Language, 13,* 293–307.

Szekeres, S., Ylvisaker, M., & Cohen, S. B. (1987). A framework for cognitive rehabilitation therapy. In M. Ylvisaker & E. M. Gobble (Eds.), *Community reentry for head injured adults* (pp. 87–136). Austin, TX: Pro-Ed.

Szekeres, S., Ylvisaker, M., & Holland, A. (1985). Cognitive rehabilitation therapy: A framework for intervention. In M. Ylvisaker (Ed.), *Head injury rehabilitation: Children and adolescents* (pp. 219– 246). Austin, TX: Pro-Ed.

Taylor, S. E. (1983). Adjustment to threatening events: A theory of cognitive adaptation. *American Psychologist, 38,* 1161–1173.

Teasdale, G., & Jennett, B. (1974). Assessment of coma and impaired consciousness: A practical scale. *Lancet, 2,* 81–84.

Thompson, C. K. (1989). Generalization in the treatment of aphasia. In L. V. McReynolds & J. E. Spradlin (Eds.), *Generalization strategies in the treatment of communication disorders* (pp. 82–115). Philadelphia: B. C. Decker.

Townsend, D. J., Carrithers, C., & Bever, T. G. (1987). Listening and reading processes in college and middle school-age readers. In R. Horowitz & S. J. Samuels (Eds.), *Comprehending oral and reading language* (pp. 217–242). New York: Academic Press.

Tromp, E., & Mulder, T. (1991). Slowness of information processing after traumatic brain injury. *Journal of Clinical and Experimental Neuropsychology, 13,* 821–830.

Trower, P., Bryant, B., & Argyle, M. (1978). *Social skills and mental health.* Pittsburgh: University of Pittsburgh Press.

Tulving, E. (1985). How many memory systems are there? *American Psychologist, 40,* 385–398.

Tupper, D. E., & Cicerone, K. D. (1990). Introduction to the neuropsychology of everyday life. In K. D. Cicerone & D. E. Tupper (Eds.), *The neuropsychology of everyday life: Assessment and basic competencies* (pp. 3–18). Boston: Kluwer Academic Publishers.

Ulatowska, H. K., Allard, L., & Chapman, S. B. (1990). Narrative and procedural discourse in aphasia. In Y. Joanette & H. H. Brownell (Eds.), *Discourse ability and brain damage: Theoretical and empirical perspectives* (pp. 180–198). New York: Springer-Verlag.

Ulatowska, H. K., Freedman-Stern, R., Weiss, D. A., Macaluso-Haynes, S., & North, A. J. (1983). Production of narrative discourse in aphasia. *Brain and Language, 19,* 317–334.

Ulatowska, H., North, A., & Macaluso-Haynes, S. (1981). Production of narrative and procedural discourse in aphasia. *Brain and Language, 13,* 345–371.

Valletutti, P. J., & Dummett, L. (1992). *Cognitive development: A functional approach.* San Diego: Singular Publishing Group.

van Dijk, T. (1977). Semantic macro-structures and knowledge frames in discourse comprehension. In M. A. Just & P. A. Carpenter (Eds.), *Cognitive processes in comprehension* (pp. 3–32). Hillsdale, NJ: Lawrence Erlbaum.

Van Zomeren, A. H. (1981). *Reaction time and attention after closed head injury.* Lisse, Switzerland: Swets and Zeitlinger.

Van Zomeren, A. H., & Brouwer, W. H. (1987). Head injury and concepts of attention. In H. S. Levin, J. Grafman, & H. M. Eisenberg (Eds.), *Neurobehavioral recovery from head injury* (pp. 398–415). New York: Oxford University Press.

Van Zomeren, A. H., Brouwer, W. H., & Deelman, B. G. (1984). Attentional deficits: The riddles of selectivity, speed, and alertness. In N. Brooks (Ed.), *Closed-head injury: Psychological, social and family consequences* (pp. 74–107). Oxford: Oxford University Press.

Varney, N. R. (1991). Iowa Collateral Head Injury Interview 1989. *Neuropsychology, 5,* 223–225.

Varney, N. R., & Menefee, L. (1993). Psychosocial and executive deficits following closed head injury: Implications for orbital frontal cortex. *Journal of Head Trauma Rehabilitation, 8*(1), 32–44.

Vogenthaler, D., Smith, K., & Goldfader, P. (1989). Head injury, a multivariate study: Predicting long-term productivity and independent living outcome. *Brain Injury, 3,* 369–386.

Wallander, J. L., Conger, A. J., & Conger, J. C. (1985). Development and evaluation of a behaviorally referenced rating system for heterosocial skills. *Behavioral Assessment, 7,* 137–153.

Warrington, E. K. (1984). *Recognition Memory Test.* Windsor: NFER-Nelson Publishing Company Ltd.

Weber, A. M. (1990). A practical clinical approach to understanding and treating attentional problems. *Journal of Head Trauma Rehabilitation, 5*(1), 73–85.

Webster, J. S., & Scott, R. R. (1983). The effects of self-instructional training on attentional deficits following head injury. *Clinical Neuropsychology, 5,* 69–74.

Wechsler, D. (1981). *Wechsler Adult Intelligence Scale—Revised.* San Antonio, TX: The Psychological Corporation.

Wechsler, D. (1987). *The Wechsler Memory Scale—Revised.* San Antonio, TX: The Psychological Corporation.

Wenzinger, K. S., Nemec, S. A., DePompei, R., & Flexer, C. (1991). The audiologist: An essential member of the rehabilitation team for traumatic brain injury. *NeuroRehabilitation, 1*(3), 41–51.

Whiteneck, G. G. (1992). Outcome evaluation and spinal cord injury. *NeuroRehabilitation, 2*(4), 31–41.

Whitman, M. (1991). Case management in head injury rehabilitation. *Rehabilitation Nursing, 16*(1), 19–22.

Whitman, S., Coonley-Hoganson R., & Desai, B. T. (1984). Comparative head trauma experience in two socioeconomically different Chicago-area communities: A population study. *American Journal of Epidemiology, 4,* 570–580.

Whitney, J. L., & Goldstein, H. (1989). Using self-monitoring to reduce disfluencies in speakers with mild aphasia. *Journal of Speech and Hearing Disorders, 54,* 576–586.

Wiemann, J. M. (1977). Explication and test of a model of communicative competence. *Human Communication Research, 3,* 195–313.

Wiig, E. (1982a). *Let's talk: Developing prosocial communication skills.* San Antonio, TX: The Psychological Corporation.

Wiig, E. (1982b). *Let's talk inventory for adolescents.* San Antonio, TX: The Psychological Corporation.

Wiig, E., & Semel, E. (1974). Development of comprehension of logicogrammatical sentences by grade school children. *Perceptual and Motor Skills, 38,* 171–176.

Wilkerson, D. L. (1992). Trends in functional assessment. (Teleconference). Rockville, MD: American Speech-Language-Hearing Association.

Willer, B. (1993). The Whatever It Takes Model. *Community Integration, 3*(3), 6–7.

Willer, B., Allen, K., Anthony, J., & Cowlan, G. (1993). *Circles of support for individuals with acquired brain injury.* Buffalo: State University of New York at Buffalo.

Willer, B., Abosh, S., & Dahmer, E. (1990). Epidemiology of disability from traumatic brain injury. In R. Wood (Ed.), *Neurobehavioral sequelae of traumatic brain injury* (pp. 18–33). New York: Taylor and Francis.

Willer, B., Allen, K., Durnan, M., & Ferry, A. (1990). Problems and coping strategies of mothers, siblings and young adult males with traumatic brain injury. *Canadian Journal of Rehabilitation, 3,* 167–173.

Williams, J. M. (1993a). Supporting families after head injury: Implications for the speech-language pathologist. *Seminars in Speech and Language, 14,* 44–60.

Williams, J. M. (1993b). Training staff for family-centered rehabilitation: Future directions in program planning. In C. J. Durgin, N. D. Schmidt, & L. J. Fryer (Eds.), *Staff development and clinical intervention in brain injury rehabilitation* (pp. 45–55). Gaithersburg, MD: Aspen Publishers.

Wilson, B. A. (1987). *Rehabilitation of memory.* New York: Guilford Press.

Wilson, B., Cockburn, J., & Baddeley, A. (1985). *Rivermead Behavioural Memory Test.* Reading, England: Thomas Valley Test Company.

Wimmer, H., & Perner, J. (1983). Beliefs about beliefs: Representation and constraining function of wrong beliefs in young children's understanding of deception. *Cognition, 13,* 103–128.

Winograd, T. (1977). A framework for understanding discourse. In M. Just & P. Carpenter (Eds.), *Cognitive processes in comprehension* (pp. 63–88). Hillsdale, NJ: Lawrence Erlbaum.

Wolfensberger, W. (1983). Social role valorization: A proposed new term for the principle of normalization. *Mental Retardation, 21,* 234–239.

Wong, S. E, Martinez-Diaz, J. A., Massel, H. K., Edelstein, B. A., Wiegand, W., Bowen, L., Bowen, L., & Liberman, R. P. (1993). Conversational skills training with schizophrenic inpatients: A study of generalization across settings and conversants. *Behavior Therapy, 24,* 285–304.

Wong, S. E., & Woolsey, J. E. (1989). Re-establishing conversational skills in overtly psychotic, chronic schizophrenic patients: Discrete trials training on the psychiatric ward. *Behavior Modification, 13,* 415–430.

Wood, R. L. (1987). *Brain injury rehabilitation: A neurobehavioral approach.* Gaithersburg, MD: Aspen.

Wood, R. L. (1988). Management of behavior disorders in a day treatment setting. *The Journal of Head Trauma Rehabilitation, 3,* 53–61.

Wood, R. L. (1990). Towards a model of cognitive rehabilitation. In R. L. Wood & I. Fussey (Eds.), *Cognitive rehabilitation in perspective* (pp. 3–24). New York: Taylor and Francis.

Wood, R. L., & Fussey, I. (1987). Computer based cognitive retraining: A controlled study. *International Disability Studies, 9,* 149–153.

Woodcock, R. W., & Johnson, M. B. (1977). *Woodcock-Johnson Psychoeducational Battery.* New York: Teachers Resources.

World Health Organization. (WHO). (1980). *International classification of impairment disabilities and handicaps.* Geneva: World Health Organization.

Wright, K. C., & DeGenaro, G. J. (1981). Supervision of the rehabilitation team. In W. G. Emener, R. S. Luck, & S. J. Smits (Eds.), *Rehabilitation administration and supervision* (pp. 253–266). Baltimore, MD: University Park Press.

Ylvisaker, M. (Ed.). (1985). *Head injury rehabilitation: Children and adolescents.* Austin, TX: Pro-Ed.

Ylvisaker, M. (1992). Communication outcome following traumatic brain injury. *Seminars in Speech and Language, 13,* 239–251.

Ylvisaker, M., Feeney, T. J., & Urbanczyk, B. (1993a). Developing a positive communication culture for rehabilitation: Communication training for staff and family members. In C. J. Durgin, N. D. Schmidt, & L. J. Fryer (Eds.), *Staff development and clinical intervention in brain injury rehabilitation* (pp. 57–86). Gaithersburg, MD: Aspen Publishers.

Ylvisaker, M., Feeney, T. J., & Urbanczyk, B. (1993b). A social-environmental approach to communication and behavior after traumatic brain injury. *Seminars in Speech and Language, 14,* 74–90.

Ylvisaker, M., & Gobble, E. M. (Eds.). (1987). *Community re-entry for head injured adults.* Austin, TX: Pro-Ed.

Ylvisaker, M., & Holland, A. (1985). Coaching, self-coaching, and rehabilitation of head injury. In D. Johns (Ed.), *Clinical management of neurogenic communicative disorders* (2nd ed.). Boston: Little, Brown and Company.

Ylvisaker, M., & Szekeres, S. F. (1989). Metacognitive and executive impairments in head-injured children and adults. *Topics in Language Disorders, 9*(2), 34–49.

Ylvisaker, M., Szekeres, S. F., Henry, K., Sullivan, D. M., & Wheeler, P. (1987). Topics in cognitive rehabilitation therapy. In M. Ylvisaker & E. M. R. Gobble (Eds.), *Community re-entry for head injured adults* (pp. 137–220). Austin, TX: Pro-Ed.

Ylvisaker, M., & Urbanczyk, B. (1990). The efficacy of speech-language pathology intervention: Traumatic brain injury. *Seminars in Speech and Language, 11,* 215–226.

Ylvisaker, M., Urbanczyk, B., & Feeney, T. J. (1992). Social skills following traumatic brain injury. *Seminars in Speech and Language, 13,* 308–322.

Yorkston, K. M., & Beukelman, D. R. (1980). An analysis of connected speech samples of aphasic and normal speakers. *Journal of Speech and Hearing Disorders, 45,* 27–36.

Zasler, N. D. (1991). Pharmacological aspects of cognitive function following traumatic brain injury. In J. S. Kreutzer & P. Wehman (Eds.), *Cognitive rehabilitation for persons with traumatic brain injury: A functional approach* (pp. 87–94). Baltimore: Paul H. Brookes Publishing Co.

Zasler, N. D. (1992). Advances in neuropharmacological rehabilitation for brain dysfunction. *Brain Injury, 6,* 1–14.

Zencius, A. H., Lane, I., & Wesolowski, M. D. (1991). Assessing and treating non-compliance in brain-injured clients. *Brain Injury, 5,* 369–374.

Zencius, A. H., Wesolowski, M. D., & Burke, W. H. (1990). A comparison of four memory strategies with traumatically brain-injured clients. *Brain Injury, 4,* 33–38.

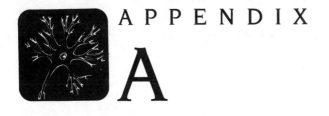

A P P E N D I X
A

Case History Form

Case History Form

NAME: _____   I.D.#: _____

DATE: _____ D.O.B.: _____   AGE: _____

PERSON(S) INTERVIEWED: _____

RELATIONSHIP: _____

MEDICAL INFORMATION

Chief Complaint: _____
_____

Circumstances leading to disability (including date, type of injury):
_____
_____
_____
_____
_____

Initial Glascow Coma Scale: _____

Length of coma: _____

Length of posttraumatic amnesia: _____

CT/MRI findings: _____

Other diagnostic findings: _____
Surgical procedures: _____

Medical complications: _____
_____

Motor deficits: _____
_____

Sensory deficits:

      Smell _____

      Taste _____

      Hearing _____

      Vision _____

      Temperature _____

      Tactile/Touch _____

      Proprioception _____

Cognitive, communicative and behavioral changes:

_____
_____
_____

Current medications:

Name	Dosage/Frequency	Reason for taking

Seizure activity: _____

Bowel and bladder concerns: _____

Dietary/nutritional concerns: _____

Appetite and weight changes: _____

Sleep habits: _____

Current medical status: _____

Preinjury medical history: _____

Medical Treatment/Rehabilitation to this point:

Facility Name/Location	Dates	Purpose

DEVELOPMENTAL/EDUCATIONAL HISTORY

Developmental milestones: _____

Highest grade completed: _____ School: _____

Additional training: _____

Premorbid learning or behavior problems/special assistance provided: _____

Best subjects: _____

Worst subjects: _____

Learning style/study habits: _____

PSYCHOSOCIAL HISTORY

Marital status: Single _____ Married _____ Divorced _____ Separated _____ Widowed _____

Preinjury living situation: _____

Current living situation: _____

Family of origin:

	Name	Occupation	Comments
Father:	_____	_____	_____
Mother:	_____	_____	_____
Siblings:	_____	_____	_____
	_____	_____	_____
	_____	_____	_____

Current Family/Support system (including friends):

Name	Age	Relationship

Premorbid history of friendships: _____
Premorbid personality, coping mechanisms: _____

Preinjury psychiatric diagnoses or treatment for mental health: _____

Substance use/abuse pattern (alcohol, illegal drugs, tobacco):
      Preinjury   _____

      Postinjury   _____

Postinjury adjustment:
      Individual   _____

Family _____

_____

WORK HISTORY_____

Job Title/Duties	Company and Location	Dates To	From

Possibility of return to previous job?   Y   N
If Yes, name/phone number of supervisor _____
Resources for job placement: _____

LEISURE INTERESTS AND ACTIVITIES, COMMUNITY INVOLVEMENT_____

List hobbies, recreational activities, social/civic groups, religious activities, music, and movie interests, volunteer work:

PreInjury: _____

_____

PostInjury: _____

_____

PREMORBID COMMUNICATION/PERSONAL STYLE_____

Primary language: _____

Extrovert vs. Introvert style: _____

Pattern of usage:

Written communication (writing letters or notes): _____

Reading: _____

Talking (phone, in person, groups): _____

Problem–solving or conflict resolution abilities: _____

FINANCIAL/LEGAL ISSUES_____

Funding source(s) for rehab and medical needs: _____

Current sources of income/assistance: _____

Legal history (Arrests/Warrants): _____

Guardianship: _____ Self _____ Other: _____

        Type of guardianship: _____ Person _____ Estate (Conservatorship)

Lawsuit: _____ pending. Explain _____

        _____ settled

Other legal concerns: _____

TRANSPORTATION

Current mode of transportation: _____
Valid driver's license: _____ Yes _____ No
Driving evaluation postinjury: _____ Yes _____ No
Means of transportation in discharge community: _____

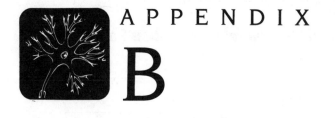

APPENDIX

B

General Behavioral Observation Form

General Behavioral Observation Form

Name: _____   Date: _____

	Within Normal Limits	Not Able to Judge	Area of Need	Comments
Attention				
Arousal				
Attention span/sustained attention				
Distractibility				
Disinhibition				
Perseveration				
Fatigibility/endurance				
Flexibility in shifting tasks				
Executive Functions/Metacognition				
Awareness of deficits/errors				
Ability to identify goals				
Spontaneous use of strategies				
Awareness of strategies used				
Ability to accept/use feedback				
Self-correction of errors/monitoring				
Rate of Processing/Responding				
Motor slowing				
Impulsivity				
Slow rate of processing/delays				
Emotional Control/Affect				
Anxiety				
Emotional lability				
Immaturity/silliness				
Anger				
Frustration tolerance				
Limited range of emotions				
Drive/Motivation				
Initiation				
Level of effort/cooperation				
Motivation for rehabilitation				
Memory				
Repetition needed				
Reauditorization				
Confabulation/Intrusions				

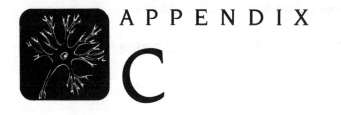

A P P E N D I X
C

Environmental Needs Assessment

Environmental Needs Assessment

Name: _____   Date: _____

Source(s) of Information: _____

LIVING/FAMILY ENVIRONMENT

Type of Setting	Current	Projected
Nursing home/subacute rehab		
Rehab facility (acute or transitional)		
Group home		
Supported living		
Independent living		
Other _____		
Activities Applicable to Individual		
Self–care		
Medication/medical condition management		
Meal planning/preparation		
Budgeting, money management		
Bill payment		
Light or routine housework		
Heavy housework		
Laundry & clothing care		
Home repairs		
Use of telephone		
Time management, scheduling		
Home safety/emergencies		
Yard work		
Child care/parenting		
Correspondence/greeting cards		
Moving arrangements		
Reading magazines/newspaper		
Watching TV/videos		
Card or board games		
Other _____		

Social Interactions
Initiation   _____
Appropriateness   _____
Responsiveness to   _____
   needs of others

Note: From "Assessment of Functional Communication" (pp. 164–167) by L. L. Hartley, 1990. In D. Tupper and K. Cicerone (Eds.), *The Neuropsychology of Everyday Life, Vol. 1: Assessment and Basic Competencies.* Boston: Kluwer Academic. Copyright 1990 by Kluwer Academic Publishers. Adapted by permission.

Individuals With Regular Contact in Living/Family Environment:

	Name	Age	Relationship
Current			
At discharge			

GENERAL COMMUNITY ENVIRONMENT

Applicable Activities/Settings	Current	Projected
Community orientation/use of map		
Mobility and safety as a pedestrian		
Use of taxi		
Use of public transportation		
Grocery shopping		
Furniture shopping		
Shopping--clothes & personal items		
Pharmacy		
Mall		
Banking/Money management		
Post Office		
Restaurants--Fast food		
Restaurants--Sit-down		
Social service agencies		
Library		
Beauty shop/Barbershop		
Doctor's offices		
Dental offices		
Rehabilitation agencies		
Religious observances		
Public telephones		
Dry cleaners		
Laudromat		
Lawyer's office/legal affairs		
Insurance companies		
Travel arrangements		
Major transportation terminals		
Support groups/social organizations		
Movie theaters		
Visiting friends in homes		
Emergencies in community		
Social interactions		

Individuals With Whom Regular Contact is Made

Name	Location	Relationship

EDUCATIONAL ENVIRONMENT

Settings
Adult basic education classes
Vocational training
High school
Community college
University
Graduate school

Activities
Study skills
Completing assignments
Turning–in assignments
Test–taking
Note–taking in class
Reading textbook
Social interactions
Written papers, letters

Current	Projected

Individuals With Whom Regular Contact is Made in These Activities

Name	Relationship

Current Educational Program
Purpose of educational program:
Major area of study:
Name of academic institution:

Courses currently taking:

Contact person:

Future Educational Plans
Purpose:

Major area of study:

Name of institution:
Courses planned:

Contact person:

WORK ENVIRONMENT

Type of Placement

Sheltered workshop
Volunteer work
Supported work
Competitive employment
Other _____

Current	Projected

Current Placement
Setting/business:

Job title and responsibilities:

Persons having regular contact/their relationship to client:

Projected Placement
Setting/business:
Job title and responsibilities:

Persons who will have regular contact with client and relationship:

Codes for Rating Level of Independence in Activities:

NA = Not applicable   V = Can do but needs verbal cues
 I = Totally independent   P = Needs minimal physical assistance
 S = Needs occasional supervision   D = Totally dependent

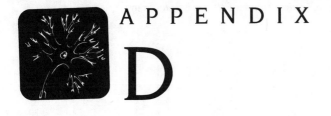

A P P E N D I X

D

Example of an Ecological Inventory

Example of an Ecological Inventory

I. RESIDENCE

ENVIRONMENT	SUB-ENVIRONMENT	ACTIVITY	SKILL	PERFORMANCE	NEEDS/COMMENTS
REHAB CENTER (PRESENT)	BEDROOM	HOUSEKEEPING	HANGING UP CLOTHES		
			MAKING UP BED		
			VACUUMING		
		SELF-CARE	DENTAL CARE		
			HAIR STYLING		
			DRESSING		
	LAUNDRY	CLOTHING CARE	SORTING CLOTHES		
			WASHING CLOTHES		
			DRYING CLOTHES		
			FOLDING CLOTHES		
	BATHROOM	HYGIENE	TOILETING		
			SHOWERING/BATHING		
	GENERAL	MEDICATION	USE OF MEDICATION		
			REFILLS OF MEDICATIONS		
		SAFETY	FIRST AID		
			FIRE DRILLS		
			AWARENESS OF DANGERS		
			JUDGMENT		
		TIME	CONCEPTS		
			MANAGEMENT OF TIME		

ENVIRONMENT	SUB-ENVIRONMENT	ACTIVITY	SKILL	PERFORMANCE	NEEDS/COMMENTS
HOME (FUTURE)		MONEY	CONCEPTS OF MONEY		
			BUDGETING		
			CARRYING MONEY SAFELY		
			WRITING CHECKS		
			USING BANK		
			STAYING WITHIN BUDGET		
			READING BILLS		
			RECONCILING STATEMENT		
	YARD	YARD MAINTENANCE	MOWING		
			RAKING		
			REMOVING TRASH		
			TRIMMING BUSHES		
	PATIO	GRILLING	USE OF GRILL		
			SAFETY		
			CLEANING		
	KITCHEN	APPLIANCES	USE OF GAS STOVE		
			USE OF ELECTRIC STOVE		
			USE OF MICROWAVE		
			USE OF DISHWASHER		
			MAINTENANCE		
			SAFETY		
	GENERAL	SOCIALIZATION	EXPRESSING NEEDS, WANTS		
			EXPRESSING FEELINGS		
			ATTENDING TO OTHERS		
			RESPONDING TO OTHERS		
			AVOIDING CONFLICTS		
			RESOLVING CONFLICTS		
			JOINING IN CONVERSATIONS		
			SHARING		
		CHILD CARE	DISCIPLINING CHILD		
			PLAYING WITH CHILD		

II. LEISURE

ENVIRONMENT	SUB-ENVIRONMENT	ACTIVITY	SKILL	PERFORMANCE	NEEDS/COMMENTS
HOME (FUTURE)	FAMILY ROOM	WATCHING TV	UNDERSTANDING NEWS		
			UNDERSTANDING WEATHER		
			READING TV GUIDE		
		MAIL	READING CARDS		
			SENDING CARDS		
			READING LETTERS		
			SENDING LETTERS		
		GAMES	PLAYING CARDS		
			BOARD GAMES		
			CROSSWORD PUZZLES		
		VIDEOTAPES	TAPING A PROGRAM		
			PLAYING VIDEOTAPE		
		NEWSPAPER	READING ARTICLES		
			READING WANT–ADS		
			READING COMICS		
			READING WEATHER		
			READING MOVIE SECTION		
			STARTING/CANCELLING		
THEATER	TICKET BOOTH	TICKET PURCHASE	WAITING IN LINE		
			READING SIGN		
			REQUESTING TICKET		
			PAYING FOR TICKET		
	CONCESSIONS	FOOD PURCHASE	WAITING TURN		
			READING SIGN		
			PLACING ORDER		
			PAYING FOR FOOD		

III. COMMUNITY

SUB-ENVIRONMENT	ACTIVITY	SKILL	PERFORMANCE	NEEDS/COMMENTS
WAL.-KCUSTOMER SERVICE	MERCHANDISE RETURN	EXPLAINING RETURN		
		REQUESTING REFUND OR EXCHANGE		
		COMPLETING FORM		
DRESSING ROOM	TRYING ON CLOTHES	LOCATING DRESSING ROOMS		
		REQUESTING ROOM		
CLOTHING DEPT.	SELECTING CLOTHES	FINDING SIZE		
		READING LABELS, TAGS		
		JUDGING QUALITY		
DR. SMWAITING ROOM OFFICE	CHECKING IN	SIGNING REGISTER		
EXAMINING ROOM	DOCTOR EXAM	STATING PROBLEM		
		FOLLOWING DIRECTIONS		
		UNDERSTANDING FINDINGS AND RECOMMENDATIONS		

IV. VOCATIONAL

ENVIRONMENT	SUB-ENVIRONMENT	ACTIVITY	SKILL	PERFORMANCE	NEEDS/COMMENTS
AMERICAN NATIONAL INSURANCE COMPANY	WORK STATION	SORTING INTER-OFFICE MAIL	READING NUMBERS ON INTEROFFICE ENVELOPES		
			SORTING BY ROUTE NUMBER INTO BINS ON DESK		
			PLACING RUBBER BAND AROUND STACK		
			PUTTING STACK INTO APPROPRIATE BOX ON CONVEYOR BELT		
	TIME CLOCK	PUNCHING CLOCK	FINDING OWN TIME CARD		
			PUNCHING IN/OUT		
			RETURNING CARD		
	BREAK TIME	GOING TO BATH-ROOM	LOCATING RESTROOM		
			TOILETING		
			CHECKING GROOMING		
		VENDING MACHINE	LOCATING MACHINE		
			PUTTING MONEY IN		
			MAKING SELECTION		
	GENERAL	TIME MANAGEMENT	TAKING BREAKS, LUNCH		
			STAYING ON TASK		

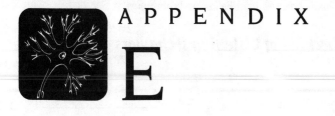

APPENDIX

E

Checklist of Listening Behaviors

Checklist of Listening Behaviors

Name: _____ Date: _____

Setting(s) Observed: _____

Indicate the frequency of the following listening behaviors in conversations or group activities.

	Almost never	Seldom	Sometimes	Often	Always	Comments
Maintains proper level of arousal						
Not easily distracted by irrelevant noises, movement						
Inhibits internal thoughts (facial expression inconsistent with speaker's message, planning what to say rather than listening)						
Maintains eye gaze towards speaker						
Refrains from doing other tasks that might distract speaker						
Indicates level of understanding through verbal or nonverbal means						
Refrains from interrupting speaker						
Shifts attention in group as speaker changes						
Waits until directions/instructions completed before starts						
Asks for clarification/repetition when unsure of message						
Follows directions without need for excessive repetition or explanation						
Comments indicate understanding of speaker's intent (asking question vs. requesting a favor, etc.)						
Initiates questions/comments relevant to topic of discussion						
Comments indicate good grasp of main ideas/critical points of discussion						
Ties comments to those of previous speaker(s)						
Comprehends paralinguistic aspects of communication (vocal tone, loudness, fluency)						
Attends to and understands nonverbal communication (body positioning, facial expression, gestures)						

Note: From *Assessment of Functional Communication* (p. 168) by L. L. Hartley, 1990. Boston: Kluwer Academic Publishers. Copyright 1990 by Kluwer Academic Publishers. Adapted by permission.

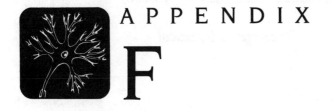

APPENDIX

F

Pragmatic Protocol

Pragmatic Protocol

NAME: _____   DATE: _____

COMMUNICATIVE   COMMUNICATIVE PARTNER'S

SETTING OBSERVED: _____   RELATIONSHIP: _____

Communicative act	Appropriate	Inappropriate	No opportunity to observe	Examples and comments
Verbal aspects				
A. Speech acts				
1. Speech act pair analysis				
2. Variety of speech acts				
B. Topic				
3. Selection				
4. Introduction				
5. Maintenance				
6. Change				
C. Turn taking				
7. Initiation				
8. Response				
9. Repair/revision				
10. Pause time				
11. Interruption/ overlap				
12. Feedback to speakers				
13. Adjacency				
14. Contingency				
15. Quantity/ conciseness				
D. Lexical selection/ use across speech acts				
16. Specificity/ accuracy				
17. Cohesion				

Communicative act	Appropriate	Inappropriate	No opportunity to observe	Examples and comments
E. Stylistic variations				
18. The varying of communicative style				
Paralinguistic aspects				
F. Intelligibility and prosodics				
19. Intelligibility and prosodics				
20. vocal intensity				
21. Vocal quality				
22. Prosody				
23. Fluency				
Nonverbal aspects				
G. Kinesics and proxemics				
24. Physical proximity				
25. Physical contacts				
26. Body posture				
27. Foot/leg and hand/arm movements				
28. Gestures				
29. Facial expression				
30. Eye gaze				

Note: From "A Clinical Appraisal of the Pragmatic Aspects of Language" by C. Prutting and D. Kirchner, 1987, *Journal of Speech and Hearing Disorders, 52,* p. 117. Copyright 1987 by American Speech-Language-Hearing Association. Reprinted by permission.

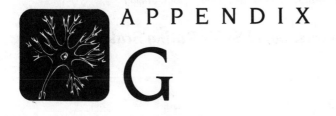

APPENDIX
G

Conversational Skills
Rating Scale

Conversational Skills Rating Scale

Person Being Rated: _____   Date: _____

Person Doing Rating: _____   Situation: _____

Rate the conversant according to how skillfully he or she used or didn't use the following communicative behaviors in the conversation, where:

1 = INADEQUATE (use was awkward, disruptive or resulted in a negative impression of communicative skills)

2 = SOMEWHAT INADEQUATE (occasionally awkward or disruptive, occasionally adequate)

3 = ADEQUATE (use was sufficient but neither very noticeable nor excellent. Produced neither positive or negative impression)

4 = GOOD (use was better than adequate but not outstanding)

5 = EXCELLENT (use was smooth, controlled, and resulted in positive impression of communicative skills)

Circle the single most accurate response for each behavior:

1 2 3 4 5   1.   Speaking rate (neither too slow nor too fast)
1 2 3 4 5   2.   Speaking fluency (avoided pauses, silences, "uh," etc.)
1 2 3 4 5   3.   Vocal confidence (neither tense nor nervous sounding)
1 2 3 4 5   4.   Articulation (language clearly pronounced and understood)
1 2 3 4 5   5.   Vocal variety (avoided monotone voice)
1 2 3 4 5   6.   Volume (neither too soft nor too loud)
1 2 3 4 5   7.   Posture (neither too closed/formal nor too open/informal)
1 2 3 4 5   8.   Lean toward partner (neither too far forward nor too far back)
1 2 3 4 5   9.   Shaking or nervous twitches (weren't noticeable)
1 2 3 4 5   10.   Unmotivated movements or fidgeting (e.g., pencil, rings, hair, fingers, etc.)
1 2 3 4 5   11.   Use of eye contact
1 2 3 4 5   12.   Facial expressiveness (neither blank nor exaggerated)
1 2 3 4 5   13.   Nodding of head in response to partner's statements
1 2 3 4 5   14.   Use of gestures to emphasize what was being said
1 2 3 4 5   15.   Smiling and/or laughing
1 2 3 4 5   16.   Use of humor and/or stories
1 2 3 4 5   17.   Asking questions
1 2 3 4 5   18.   Encouragements or agreements (encouraged partner to talk)
1 2 3 4 5   19.   Speaking about partner or partner's interests (involved partner as topic of conversation)
1 2 3 4 5   20.   Speaking about self (didn't talk too much about self/own interests)
1 2 3 4 5   21.   Expression of personal opinions (neither too passive or aggressive)
1 2 3 4 5   22.   Initiation of new topics
1 2 3 4 5   23.   Maintenance of topics and follow up comments
1 2 3 4 5   24.   Interruption of partner's speaking turns
1 2 3 4 5   25.   Use of time speaking relative to partner

For the next five items, rate the person's overall conversational performance:

(26)   Poor Conversationalist   1 2 3 4 5   Excellent Conversationalist
(27)   Socially Unskilled   1 2 3 4 5   Socially Skilled
(28)   Incompetent Interactant   1 2 3 4 5   Competent Interactant
(29)   Inappropriate Interactant   1 2 3 4 5   Appropriate Interactant
(30)   Ineffective Interactant   1 2 3 4 5   Effective Interactant

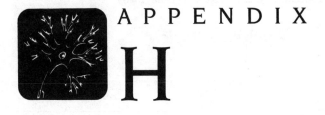

APPENDIX

H

Analysis of Topic

Analysis of Topic

Name: _____   Date: _____
Setting: _____   Partner: _____
Length of Time: _____

| | Frequency | | Comments |
	Client	Partner	
Topic Initiation/Introduction			
Subject matter			
New–appropriate topic			
Related–appropriate			
Reintroduced topic			
Participant orientation			
Self–oriented			
Other–oriented			
Relationship–oriented			
Communicative intent			
Obliges			
Informatives			
Topic Maintenance			
Response to an open–ended question			
Acknowledgement			
Request for more information on topic			
Addition of new, related information			
Clarification of own information			
Request for repair/clarification			
Repetition of old information			
Agreement/disagreement			
Topic shading			
Other _____			
Topic Disruptions			
Noncoherent topic change			
Ambiguous or incomplete turn			
Reintroduction–inappropriate			
Irrelevant utterance			
Multiple topic initiation			
Talking to self			
Evasion of question			
No response			
Other _____			

Note : Based on material from Bedrosian (1985, 1993) and Mentis and Prutting (1991).

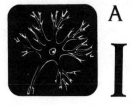

A P P E N D I X
I

Futures Planning

Futures Planning

Name: _____   Date: _____

Others Providing Input:

Name	Relationship

MAJOR LIFE EXPERIENCES, THEMES

_____

_____

_____

_____

_____

_____

_____

_____

CIRCLE OF SUPPORT (FAMILY, FRIENDS, PEERS, PAID STAFF, ETC.)

_____

_____

_____

_____

_____

_____

_____

_____

IMPORTANT PLACES (LIVING, WORK, LEISURE)

_____

_____

_____

_____

_____

_____

WHAT YOU ENJOY

LIKES	DISLIKES

CURRENT CHOICES

MADE BY YOU	MADE BY OTHERS

WHAT IS THE DESIRED FUTURE?

Home	
Work	
School	
Community	
People	

Recreation	
Legal	
Medical/ Rehab	

YOUR STRENGTHS	OBSTACLES TO OVERCOME

ACTION PLAN

Action Needed	Person(s) Responsible	Target Completion Date

Comments/Follow-up Needed: _____

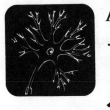

APPENDIX
J

Minimal Cognitive-Communication Competencies

Minimal Cognitive-Communication Competencies

Name:_____   Date:_____

LISTENING/LANGUAGE COMPREHENSION

The individual will:

____ understand vocabulary/concepts needed in daily living, work, leisure, or school activities
        ____ identify objects, time, and numbers when named
        ____ identify objects when described
____ comprehend simple Yes/No questions concerning general knowledge and personal history
____ understand and answer wh- questions (who, what, when, where, why) correctly
____ comprehend sentences/questions that express complex logico-grammatical relationships (i.e., comparative, spatial, temporal, passive, and familial relationships)
____ obtain important information from spoken messages
____ follow complex three-step commands
        ____ follow directions concerning a spatial route (both on map and in real-life situation)
        ____ follow directions to produce a written output
        ____ follow directions to produce a product/craft
        ____ follow directions to perform a series of actions
____ comprehend and remember main ideas and supporting details of a paragraph or conversation
____ comprehend main ideas in a small group discussion
____ detect speaker's purpose (e.g., to ask favor, to inform, to command)
____ make inferences or draw conclusions
____ distinguish fact from opinion
____ evaluate a speaker's argument
____ recognize propaganda (information versus persuasion)
____ discriminate relevant versus irrelevant information
____ realize when important aspects of message or story are missing
____ demonstrate general characteristics of a good listener (eye contact, avoid interruption, signal level of understanding, pay attention)
____ monitor own comprehension and ask for repetition or clarification when needed

LANGUAGE PRODUCTION/CONVERSATIONAL SKILLS

The individual will:

____ obtain listener's attention before speaking
____ use grammatically intact sentences and questions
____ retrieve words to express ideas precisely and accurately, without use of vague, ambiguous, or low informational words
____ use language for a variety of communication intents (speech acts, social skills)
____ express clear communicative intent to listener
____ sequence steps or organize the content in a logical manner
____ express content without excessive dysfluencies (part or whole word repetitions, revisions, and filled pauses) or silent pauses
____ use social rituals
____ initiate and maintain a conversation

_____ select appropriate topics and times for conversation
_____ ask clear, relevant and socially appropriate questions
_____ provide accurate and complete answers to questions
_____ persuade others and respond appropriately to persuasion
_____ express and respond to feelings
_____ express opinions and points of view with defending evidence
_____ tell stories of past, present, or future events
_____ provide relevant information that is sufficient in quantity to convey ideas clearly
    (without excessive details, personal experience/evaluation, or irrelevant comments)
_____ give clear oral directions to others
_____ take turns speaking and listening, without interrupting other person
_____ recognize when communication breakdown has occurred and repair through
    repetition, revision, or clarification
_____ use nonverbal communication, paralinguistic features appropriate for message and
    social setting (formal, informal, dealing with peers vs. supervisors, work vs. social
    setting)
_____ use communication style appropriate for his/her age level
_____ interact with peers, family and supervisors in a way that indicates sensitivity to their
    feelings
_____ link the meanings of sentences or turns together
_____ summarize messages or events to facilitate mutual understanding or share
    information

VERBAL INTEGRATION AND REASONING

The individual will:

_____ understand and use abstract language forms
    _____ comprehend and use idiomatic expressions and proverbs
    _____ comprehend metaphors, fables, and jokes
    _____ detect absurdities
_____ use language to solve safety and interpersonal problems
    _____ identify problematic situations
    _____ generate alternative solutions to problem situations
    _____ consider possible outcomes of each solution
    _____ select and implement best solution
    _____ evaluate outcome of problem solving
    _____ resolve interpersonal conflicts by stating and explaining/describing differences
        of opinion
_____ use language for reasoning
    _____ understand and express cause-effect relationships
    _____ understand and express if-then situations
    _____ compare and contrast ideas, situations, objects
    _____ understand and express both sides of an issue (pros & cons)

Note: From "A Functional Approach to the Cognitive-Communicative Deficits of Closed Head Injured Clients" by L. L. Hartley and A. Griffith, 1988, _Tejas: Texas Journal of Audiology and Speech Pathology, 14_(2), p. 42. Copyright by author. Adapted by permission.

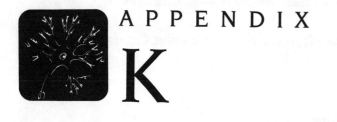

APPENDIX

K

Functional Communication Goals

Functional Communication Goals

<u>DOMAIN I: HOME</u>

A.   Personal Health Care and Safety

-- States and writes own name, address, phone number, nearest relative, and his or her
    phone number
-- If not independent, asks for assistance in toileting, dressing, grooming in appropriate
    manner
-- Reports when feeling sick, indicates problem
-- Calls emergency numbers and communicates problem, name, and address
-- Reads and follows labels on prescriptions or over-the-counter medicines
-- States purpose of common over-the-counter medicines (e.g., aspirin, Tylenol, rubbing
    alcohol, cold medicines, antibiotic cream)
-- Understands weather bulletins
-- Understands facts versus opinions concerning health, nutrition and illness treatment
    issues
- Reports doctor's findings or recommendations to significant other

B.   Family Life and Social Interactions

-- Uses and responds to greetings and farewells
-- Uses polite social rituals (please, thank-you, excuse me, etc.)
-- Introduces others
-- Initiates conversation with family and friends
-- Makes and responds to requests for actions or things
-- Gives and responds to compliments
-- Indicates feelings (happy, sad, tired, lonely, etc.) or disapproval
-- Asks wh- questions
-- Attends to and answers questions using appropriate manner and language for the
    partner
-- Offers assistance
-- Asks permission
-- Asks for repetition or clarification when doesn't understand
-- Remembers and expresses feelings regarding major life events of friends and family
    (birthday, holidays, graduation, death in family)
-- Deals with problems with neighbors appropriately
-- Responds appropriately to salespeople, solicitors
-- Recognizes problems, generates solutions, and selects appropriate solution
-- Tells stories, jokes, and anecdotes in informal settings
-- Asks for a date
-- Expresses values, concerns, and opinions to family members and friends
-- Explains unfamiliar task or chore to others thoroughly, with supporting nonverbal
    communication
-- Discusses differences in opinion regarding household or child-rearing
    responsibilities with spouse
-- Summarizes phone call discussion for family member
-- Gives directions to house or apartment for someone coming to visit

C.   Use of Memory Aids/Orientation

-- Tells time
-- Reads daily schedule
-- Reads calendar
-- Writes appointments on calendar
-- Writes and uses personal phone list
-- Writes and uses journal notes in organized manner
-- Writes and uses errand list
-- Writes and uses shopping lists
-- Writes and uses personal information sheet
-- Uses maps
-- Plans leisure activities

D.   Leisure Activities--Indoors

   -- Understands main points of TV programs or news broadcasts
   -- Summarizes what has done, seen, read, or heard in leisure activities
   -- Explains how to play a game or conduct activity to a friend or family member
   -- Arranges meeting a friend
   -- Invites friends to house
   -- Plans dinner for friends
   -- Invites friend or family member to play cards or board games
   -- Initiates listening to favorite music
   -- Requests favorite music
   -- Rents movies
   -- Plays word games (crossword puzzles, word searches)
   -- Reads books or magazines for pleasure
   -- Comprehends instructions for creative crafts (woodworking, ceramics, needlepoint, macrame) or art
   -- Communicates with friends over telephone
   -- Initiates and maintains conversation with friends in-person
   -- Writes letters
   -- Cares for pets/plants

E.   Housekeeping and Maintenance

   -- Reads and complies with labels on cleaning products
   -- Reads and uses checklist if needed to complete housekeeping duties
   -- Reads directions for putting together furniture, toy
   -- Reads and follows carefully directions on insecticides
   -- Measures with ruler
   -- Weighs self
   -- Reads simple contracts for services
   -- Arranges for maintenance with landlord or appropriate service person
   -- Explains malfunction or way wants repair done to service person
   -- Reads and follows directions for use and care of appliances
   -- Understands suggestions for preventive maintenance given by plumber, appliance or heating/air conditioning repairman

F.   Meal Planning and Preparation

   -- Writes and reads grocery list
   -- Reads labels and nutritional information on packages of food
   -- Follows directions on packages of food and other products
   -- Reads cookbook (table of contents, index)
   -- Reads and follows recipes
   -- Demonstrates safe use of cooking utensils and appliances
   -- Plans nutritional meals

G.   Use of Telephone

   -- Looks up phone numbers in white pages
   -- Uses yellow pages to find names, numbers of various businesses
   -- Keeps list of important phone numbers in memory aid and uses it
   -- Dials numbers correctly
   -- Speaks with appropriate articulation, rate, and volume to be understood
   -- Selects language that will get point across, with courtesy
   -- Understands response of other person
   -- Gives or takes directions to a location
   -- Takes phone message accurately for self or others
   -- Leaves a clear message for a person (when to return call)
   -- Leaves clear, concise message on answering machine
   -- Uses pay phone
   -- Places a direct long-distance call
   -- Places a credit card or collect long-distance call
   -- Initiates use of phone with others at appropriate level of acquaintance
   -- Takes into consideration time zones when places long-distance phone calls
   -- Knows how to dial for directory assistance, when needed
   -- Can write spoken phone number down accurately and legibly

Purposes of phone calls:

-- Arranges appointments for haircuts, dentist, doctor, and so on
-- Cancels or changes appointments/meeting times, when appropriate
-- Calls work if late or sick
-- Knows emergency number, when to use 911, and can give correct information over phone
    in emergency situation
-- Knows how to handle phone calls regarding apartment or house (i.e., to plumber,
    electrician, utilities, landlord)
-- Makes reservations for travel (bus, taxi, airlines, hotel, etc.)
-- Makes reservations at restaurant
-- Orders pizza to be delivered
-- Obtains information about goods or services
-- Obtains information about hours of operation
-- Obtains information about schedules (bus, movies, planes)
-- Calls for taxi and gives correct location
-- Calls friend and invites for visit or arranges a meeting
-- Gives directions to own home
-- Calls to connect or disconnect phone, gas, electricity, water

H.   Spoken or Written Messages

-- Obtains critical information (who, what, when, where, why, how) from a message
-- Recognizes when critical information missing
-- Expresses wh- information in clear form to others, both orally and in writing
-- Asks for modification of input, if needed (slow down, spell a word, write it)
-- Asks for repetition or clarification, if needed

I.   Correspondence

-- Reads and understands greeting cards
-- Addresses envelope
-- Writes thank--you notes when appropriate
-- Sends greeting cards to friends and family
-- Writes personal letters to friends and family
-- Comprehends letters received
-- Writes business letters that express intent clearly, to the point, and in a manner that is
    likely to accomplish purpose (obtain information, inquire about job, register complaint,
    order a product, change address or name, inform congress member)
-- Uses dictionary to look up spelling, pronunciation, or meaning

J.   Use of Newspaper

-- Reads want-ads to look for job
-- Writes and places want-ad (e.g., garage sale, sell furniture)
-- Reads TV guide
-- Reads store ads
-- Reads entertainment (movies) section
-- Uses index to paper
-- Reads weather section
-- Obtains main ideas and supporting details from newspaper articles and comics

K.   Child Care

-- Expresses approval of child's activity, performance
-- Gives appropriate verbal and nonverbal praise, reward for child's good behavior
-- Expresses disapproval of child's behavior through appropriate means, at appropriate
    level of disapproval
-- Explains desired behavior to child
-- Explains new task or chore to child with supporting nonverbal communication
-- Gives directions for game
-- Plays games with child, including verbal play such as chants, rhymes, and songs
-- Reads books to child
-- Expresses sympathy and comfort to child when hurt or upset
-- Teaches child how to handle emergencies

-- Recognizes when child does not understand instructions or situation
-- Initiates and maintains conversation with child about past, present or future events
-- Gives child choices regarding clothing, food, activities, when appropriate
-- Teaches child about nutrition
-- Explains to child about safety (playgrounds, bicycle, strangers, street)
-- Assists the child in homework
-- Expresses values and feelings to child
-- Explains financial/money issues that are developmentally appropriate
-- Answers child's questions so that child understands
-- Asks questions of child
-- Listens attentively to child's talk
-- Gives reasons for a family rule or why child should or should not do something
-- Gives clear, step-by-step directions
-- Makes requests for actions in indirect language, when appropriate

DOMAIN II: COMMUNITY

A. Mobility (office buildings, transportation terminals, streets)

-- Understands signs (buildings, streets, roadways, buses)
-- Reads directories inside buildings
-- Reads maps (finds places on map, plans route to get to a certain place)
-- Uses scale to determine distances and then predict time needed
-- Reads bus schedules, route information
-- Gives others directions to his or her place of residence, job location, or major building in community
-- Writes clear directions to another location
-- Asks for directions (to bus stop, postal office, hospital, nearest shopping center when needed
-- Responds appropriately to conversation with strangers
-- Initiates interactions as appropriate to obtain information or for conversation
-- Gives destination to taxi driver

B. Community Safety

-- States what should do if lost
-- States what to do when needs to locate facility or bus stop
-- States what to do if gets on wrong bus
-- States what to do in case of fire or injury in community
-- Identifies hazards (water on floor, large cracks in sidewalk)
-- States what to do when approached by stranger on street
-- Identifies own medical problems and what to do if experiences problem in community

C. Shopping (grocery store, department store, discount store)

-- Reads and uses information from ads
-- Writes check at check-out register
-- Reads and compares prices of items
-- Understands amount of money spoken by cashier or reads printout
-- Understands labels on clothing/goods/food (size, quantity, price, product name, contents, care of product, nutritional information)
-- Asks for assistance in store when needed (finding a particular product, size, or location of section of store)
-- Reads signs over aisles, sections of store
-- Determines category for item on grocery list (e.g., spaghetti would be under pasta)
-- Inquires about time store closes/opens
-- Inquires about store's policy on taking checks, credit cards, return of items
-- Asks about gift wrapping, asks for gift wrapping or box
-- Explains about defective or unwanted merchandise for return to clerk and asks for refund
-- Asks about care of certain item (boots, sweater, pet)
-- Gives reason for not wanting to buy a particular item
-- Reads signs in store that indicate location of items
-- Uses vending, change-making machines

-- Uses a mail order catalog and fills out order form
-- Writes and reads shopping list for clothing and personal items
-- Reads and understands warranties for products

D.   Budgeting and Banking (bank, savings and loan)

-- Selects bank based on information regarding costs, services, location
-- Reads and understands items on bills
-- Writes checks and records them in checkbook
-- Sends off check to pay bill at proper time
-- Fills out deposit/withdrawal forms, endorses check
-- Knows what to say to open bank account, make deposit or withdrawal, close account, transfer money
-- Knows who to call to inquire about account with bank
-- Reads statements from bank
-- Sets up files for receipts and paid bills
-- Deals with solicitors, salespeople
-- Reads and follows directions on ATM machine
-- Balances checkbook
-- Reads and fills in loan application forms
-- Reads simple tax forms or seeks help in completing
-- Writes monthly budget to plan expenses

E.   Other Community Activities

-- Reads menus, orders food
-- Asks for receipt/ticket/check (restaurant, movies, ride) when appropriate
-- Understands amount of money said by cashier
-- Reads instructions on games, machines
-- Obtains stamps or other items at postoffice
-- Mails a package at postoffice
-- Tells receptionist name, person with whom has an appointment, time of appointment
-- Tells barber/stylist how to cut hair
-- Asks for location of restroom, elevator

Possible Settings in Community:

Library	Fast Food Restaurant
Movie Theater	Concerts
Laundromat	Plays
Furniture store	Clubs
Post Office	Religious Services
Sit-Down Restaurant	Museums
Barber/Beauty Parlor	Parties
Health Care Facilities	Weddings
Cafeteria	Funerals

F.   Medical Care

-- Makes appointments and writes them down on calendar
-- Describes illness, symptoms, or accident thoroughly to doctor or dentist
-- Understands directions from doctor or dentist regarding medication and home care
-- Writes down next appointment on calendar
-- Recognizes a prescription and knows procedures for getting it filled
-- Reads and follows labels on medicines
-- Reads and fills in medical history forms
-- Reads and fills in insurance forms

G.   Making Independent Living Arrangements

-- Asks appropriate sources (friend, co-workers) about where to begin search
-- Looks in want-ads and yellow pages for names of places in that area (use of map, if needed)
-- Calls places to determine costs, availability, facilities, features
-- Writes down information in organized manner for comparison

-- Reads and completes application for rent
-- Reads and understands lease agreement
-- Arranges utilities (electricity, phone, gas, water)
-- Makes moving arrangements
-- Asks about and obtains household insurance
-- Reads insurance policy
-- Fills out change-of-address forms with Post Office

H. Citizen Advocate

-- Completes voter registration card
-- Reads information regarding political issues
-- Asks for location of polls
-- Uses inoffensive language and nonverbal communication when expresses political views
    or opinions to friends, governmental agencies, or civic organizations
-- Understands ballot when voting
-- Distinguishes between fact and opinion in newscasts, political messages
-- Makes a complaint to appropriate agency
-- Writes letter supporting legislation to politicians

DOMAIN III: WORK

A. Job Seeking Skills

-- Completes job application
-- Makes follow-up calls to set up interview
-- Writes resume
-- Writes letters inquiring about jobs
-- Responds completely and appropriately to typical job interview questions (e.g., personal
    history, skills and abilities, work history, education, interpersonal relationships, career
    goals or plans, questions about job)
-- Makes follow-up call after interview

B. General Job Skills

-- Calls in when sick or late
-- Follows daily schedule/routine
-- Follows spoken or written directions as given
-- Initiates next task without prompting
-- Takes phone messages, if appropriate
-- Identifies when assistance is needed/communicates need to appropriate person
-- Expresses feelings regarding job conditions to supervisor in appropriate manner
-- Copes with frustrations and anger in positive manner
-- Uses appropriate persuasive strategies
-- Responds to interactions from supervisor, co-workers, customers in appropriate manner
-- Asks customer if they need assistance (if appropriate)
-- Selects appropriate topic, time, and duration of conversation
-- Maintains appropriate eye contact, volume, tone of voice
-- Accepts correction/criticism from supervisor/co-workers
-- Reads job-related manuals, policies, signs
-- Responds to anger appropriately
-- Makes complaint in appropriate manner
-- Able to problem solve in work situations
-- Explains specific job requirements and job processes or techniques
-- Gives clear and concise report of events on job
-- Gives directions in clear and organized manner
-- Expresses and defends point of view, opinion
-- Asks questions on appropriate topics in manner that facilitates cooperation
-- Understands and describes opposing points of view
-- Writes reports when required

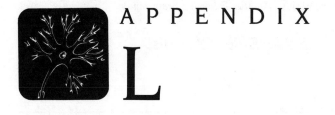

APPENDIX

L

Social Skills Checklist

Social Skills Checklist

Name: _____

RITUALS

_____ Greets others
_____ Expresses farewells
_____ Uses polite expressions
_____ Introduces self
_____ Introduces others
_____ Responds to introductions
_____ Starts conversation
_____ Maintains conversation through turn-taking strategies
_____ Closes conversation

REQUESTING INFORMATION

_____ Requests/asks name, phone number, address of someone
_____ Requests/asks location of objects, belongings
_____ Requests/asks location, time of event
_____ Requests/asks opening/closing times
_____ Requests/asks preferences or wants
_____ Requests/asks availability of product/service
_____ Requests/asks cost of product/service
_____ Requests/asks for appointment
_____ Requests repetition or clarification
_____ Asks open-ended (wh-) questions
_____ Asks yes/no questions

GIVING INFORMATION

_____ Tells own name, phone number, address
_____ Tells location of belonging or necessities
_____ Tells location and time of events
_____ Tells preferences or wants
_____ Tells name of medications taken
_____ Tells pertinent personal medical history
_____ Tells own personal strengths and weaknesses
_____ Leaves appropriate phone messages
_____ Tells height and weight, sizes, physical features
_____ Tells of past experiences, story heard
_____ Tells of ongoing event
_____ Tells future plans/goals
_____ Describes symptoms of illness, medical condition

CONTROLLING

_____ Gives instructions or directions on
            _____ how to get to a certain location
            _____ how to make a certain design or project
            _____ how to make a food dish
            _____ how to perform a series of activities
                        (game, craft, etc.)
_____ Invites friend, suggesting time and place for a meeting
_____ Asks for permission
_____ Gives permission
_____ Asks for reasons
_____ Tells reasons
_____ Asks for favor, action or assistance
_____ Responds to request for favor or assistance
_____ Responds to offers of assistance
_____ Offers assistance

_____Offers to share something
_____Makes a complaint or criticizes
_____Responds to complaint or criticism
_____Asks for intentions
_____Responds to requests for intentions
_____Asks to discontinue actions
_____Gives opinion or beliefs
_____Tries to persuade/convince others
_____Responds to persuasion/peer pressure, solicitation
_____Asks for contractual terms
_____Asks for changes in contractual terms
_____Resolves conflicts through negotiation
_____Deals with contradictory messages

SHARING FEELINGS

_____Expresses appreciation or thanks
_____Expresses agreement or approval
_____Expresses disagreement or disapproval
_____Gives a compliment
_____Apologizes
_____Accepts apology
_____Expresses affection
_____Expresses positive feelings and attitudes
_____Expresses negative feelings and attitudes
_____Responds to anger
_____Expresses emotional support/empathy
_____Responds to teasing
_____Solicits feelings of others
_____Expresses sympathy
_____Offers congratulations

Note: Based on material from Goldstein et al. (1980), Wiig (1982a), and Wood (1977).

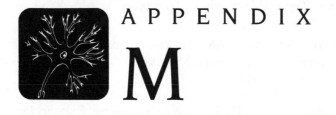

APPENDIX

M

Functional Treatment Materials Sources

Angle, D. K., & Buxton, J. M. (1991). *Community living skills workbook for the head injured adult.* Gaithersburg, MD: Aspen Publishers.

DiKengil, A., & Kaye, M. (1992). *Building functional social skills: Group activities for adults.* Tucson, AZ: Communication Skill Builders.

Hahn, S. E., & Klein, E. (1989). *Focus on function.* Tucson, AZ: Communication Skill Builders.

Holland, S., & Ward, C. (1990). *Assertiveness: A practical approach.* Bicester, Great Britain: Winslow Press.

Johnson, R. P., & Orichowskyj, R. M. (1993). *Out in the world: A community living skills manual.* Bisbee, AZ: Imaginart.

Kovich, K. M., & Bermann, D. E. (1988). *Head Injury: A guide to functional outcomes in occupational therapy.* Gaithersburg, MD: Aspen Publishers.

Lazzari, A. (1990). *Just for adults.* East Moline, IL: LinguiSystems.

Lazzari, A., & Peters, P. (1989). *Handbook of exercises for language processing: Volume 3: Concepts, paraphrasing, critical thinking, social language.* East Moline, IL: LinguiSystems.

Macro Systems (1988, 1989). *Social skills on the job: A transition to the workplace for students with special needs.* Circle Pines, MN: American Guidance Service.

McCart, W. (1989). *Learning to listen.* Cambridge, MA: Educators Publishing Services.

O'Hara, C. C., & Harrell, M. (1991). *Rehabilitation with brain injury survivors: An empowerment approach.* Gaithersburg, MD: Aspen Publishers.

Schumaker, J. B., Hazel, J. S., & Pederson, C. S. (1988). *Social skills for daily living.* Circle Pines, MN: American Guidance Service.

Schwartz, N., & McKinley, N. L. (1984). *Daily communication: Strategies for the language disordered adolescent.* Eau Claire, WI: Thinking Publications.

Sohlberg, M. M., Perlewitz, P. G., Johansen, A., Schultz, J., Johnson, L., & Hartry, A. (1993). *Improving pragmatic skills in persons with head injury.* Tucson, AZ: Communication Skill Builders.

Stiefel, B. (1987). *On my own with language.* East Moline, IL: Lingui-Systems.

Walker, H., Todis, B., Holmes, D., & Horton, G. (1988). *The access program.* Austin, TX: Pro-Ed.

Addresses

American Guidance Service
Circle Pines, MN 55014-1796

Aspen Publishers
200 Orehard Ridge Drive
Gaithersburg, MD 20878

Communication Skill Builders
3830 E. Bellevue
P.O. Box 42050-CS4
Tucson, AZ 85733

Educators Publishing Service, Inc.
31 Smith Place
Cambridge, MA 02138-1000

Imaginart
307 Arizona Street
Bisbee, AZ 85603

LinguiSystems, Inc.
3100 4th Avenue
P.O. Box 747
East Moline, IL 61244-0747

National Council of Teachers
of English
1111 Kenyon Road
Urbana, IL 61801

Pro-Ed
8700 Shoal Creek Boulevard
Austin, TX 78757-6897

Speech Communication
Association
5105 Backlick Road, Suite E
Annadale, VA 22003

Thinking Publications
P.O. Box 163
Eau Claire, WI 54702-0163

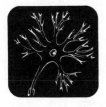

Index